AUDREY COHEN COLLEGE

Y0-CVI-783

HV
675.72
S28
1991

Saving children

APR 13 1995

JAN 02 1995

COLLEGE FOR HUMAN SERVICES
LIBRARY
345 HUDSON STREET
NEW YORK, N.Y. 10014

Saving Children

Saving Children

A GUIDE TO INJURY PREVENTION

Modena Hoover Wilson
Susan P. Baker
Stephen P. Teret
Susan Shock
James Garbarino

New York   Oxford
OXFORD UNIVERSITY PRESS
1991

Oxford University Press

Oxford New York Toronto
Delhi Bombay Calcutta Madras Karachi
Petaling Jaya Singapore Hong Kong Tokyo
Nairobi Dar es Salaam Cape Town
Melbourne Auckland

and associated companies in
Berlin Ibadan

Copyright © 1991 by Oxford University Press, Inc.

Published by Oxford University Press, Inc.,
200 Madison Avenue, New York, New York 10016

Oxford is a registered trademark of Oxford University Press

All rights reserved. No part of this publication may be reproduced,
stored in a retrieval system, or transmitted, in any form or by any means,
electronic, mechanical, photocopying, recording, or otherwise,
without the prior permission of Oxford University Press.

Library of Congress Cataloging-in-Publication Data
Saving children : a guide to injury prevention / by Modena Hoover
Wilson . . . [et al.].
p. cm. Includes bibliographical references.
ISBN 0-19-506115-2
1. Children's accidents—United States—Prevention.
2. Traffic safety and children—United States.
3. Home accidents—United States—Prevention.
4. School accidents—United States—Prevention.
I. Wilson, Modena Hoover.
HV675.72.S28 1991 363.1′0083—dc20 90-7279

1 3 5 7 9 8 6 4 2

Printed in the United States of America
on acid-free paper

FOREWORD

Nothing under the sun is accidental.
—Gotthold Ephraim Lessing, 1772

No great blueprint, but rather a series of incidents—coincidence—often determines our career paths. Yogi Berra said, "When you come to a fork in the road, take it." It was that way for me, choosing both pediatrics as a career and injury control as a major professional interest. By chance, the late summer of 1971 found me on my first clinical rotation in medical school assigned to pediatrics at Cooper Hospital in a very hot and humid Camden, New Jersey. Pediatrics at Cooper was busy, even chaotic, with lots of pneumonia, diarrhea, asthma, and diabetes. By mid-September, the enthusiasm of my teachers (and optimistic prognosis for most of my patients) cemented my decision to become a pediatrician.

My first day at Cooper, I met Billie, a blond, 9-year-old boy from East Camden who had been the victim of an "unfortunate accident." Billie had been climbing a tree. He fell out of the tree, landing belly-first across the top edge of an iron fence. He had been admitted to the surgical service for management of his abdominal injuries.

Five summers later my wife, Ruth, and I found ourselves in an equally hot and humid Baltimore, Maryland. I had completed medical school and my pediatric residency. Ruth and I had each been awarded traineeships to spend a year at The Johns Hopkins School of Public Health. Ruth's academic advisor, Timothy Baker, suggested she take a course taught by his wife, Susan Baker, entitled "Issues in Injury Control"—hardly the standard fare in a school of public *health*. Ruth agreed to register for the course on the condition that she could convince her husband to take the course with her. From the first day of class, it was clear that both the teacher and the subject were to be something out of the ordinary. (Susan Baker's good preparation and attention to detail extended to her memorizing by the end of the first session the names of every student.) In 12 sessions, we learned a new way of thinking about injuries, adopting the tools (and the skepticism) of our teacher, the epidemiologist. We learned that injuries occurred neither randomly nor capriciously but rather in predictable patterns determined by recognizable risk factors. As with infectious diseases, one's likelihood of being injured — in an automobile crash, in a swimming pool, or by gunfire — was determined largely by the quantity and quality of one's exposure to sources of harmful energy coupled with the physical means (e.g., a dashboard) to transmit that energy to the body. And, as with infectious diseases, populations could be protected from injury not only by limiting their exposure but also by immunization. (This book tells you how!) The subject came alive with Professor Baker's liberal use of instructive example and pertinent detail, drawn from her own pioneering work as well as from the then sparse literature on injury prevention. Most importantly, we learned that we were in possession of the theory, the technology, and the resources to both predict and prevent injuries, and in so doing, could, with the standard tools of preventive medicine, reverse the major public health challenge of industrialized countries.

Since medical school, I had not thought much about Billie. Billie had died, somewhat unexpectedly, after 23 days in the hospital. Now, after 5 years, I could put his tragedy into a new context. I thought about the many factors and links in the chain of events that led to his fatal injury: the height of the tree, the design of the fence, the recreational opportunities available to Billie in East Camden, the availability of emergency services, and the lack of availability of a designated pediatric trauma center. Injury prevention was not a subject taught in medical school in 1977. It is not often taught now. In any event, my studies in Baltimore served well to stimulate my thinking as a physician and to complement my clinical training.

This book is an effort to draw people into the kind of thinking necessary to prevent needless injury to our children. The goal is to apply currently available knowledge by enlisting decision makers as part of an ad hoc multidisciplinary team. In the 13 years since I left Baltimore, Professor Baker has attracted to Hopkins an impressive array of individuals to study, teach, and advocate a safer environment for our children. The Johns Hopkins Injury Prevention Center, now directed by Stephen Teret, is characterized not only by its enthusiasm and competence but also by its promotion of a multidisciplinary approach, as evidenced in this book: Modena Wilson is a pediatrician; Susan Baker, an epidemiologist; Stephen Teret, an attorney; Susan Shock, a writer and editor. They are joined by child-development specialist James Gabarino, president of Chicago's highly regarded Erikson Institute, to lay out for professionals a blueprint for identifying and weakening the links in the chain of circumstances that lead to childhood injuries.

Saving Children underscores the point that just as there are multiple factors predisposing to injury, there are multiple countermeasures from which to choose. Automobiles can be made more crashworthy, society can become less tolerant of drunken drivers, and we can become more competent in providing emergency and rehabilitative services to crash victims. Just as the patient with asthma is provided a combination of drugs which act synergistically to prevent wheezing, so too injuries can be prevented by a combination of strategies used together. Patients often need and benefit from multiple consultants, and injury prevention can likewise benefit from a variety of experts. The authors state that it would be hard to imagine an adult whose professional decisions do not impact upon children's risk of injury. As one reads, one is persuaded how true that is.

Stemming the epidemic of childhood injuries will take the best thinking and best decision making of a wide range of adults. We are advancing from the old and narrow arsenal of remedies such as telling people to "be careful" and handing them a pamphlet. We no longer take satisfaction in assigning blame. That is not how we learned to prevent measles and whooping cough. That is not how we will prevent injuries.

It is summer 1990, and I again think of Billie. Perhaps it is because I realize that even medical students graduating today are still largely ignorant of the principles of injury prevention. The same is true for students of law, engineering, business, architecture, and many other fields. This lack of training is a continuing disservice to our children.

Perhaps I now think of 9-year-old Billie because of 9-year-old Daniel, who lives at my house. There are about 3.5 million 9-year-olds in the United States today; about 700 of them will die in the next 12 months, 450 of them from injuries. (Motor vehicles will claim about 200; drownings, 65 or 70; 45 will succumb to fire and smoke; and at least 30 will die from gunfire.) Incredibly, we are in a much better position scientifically and technologically to prevent these injury deaths than the deaths from other causes. Unfortunately, there is a wide gap between what is known about injury prevention and what is taught to those in a position to apply that knowledge.

Saving Children attempts to bridge the gap between "know-how" and application of that knowledge. It is a book with a message. But it is also an intellectual refreshment of the first order, a brainstorming session filled with hundreds of injury-prevention strategies, dozens of which can be influenced by your decisions as a state legislator, a volunteer firefighter, a delivery room nurse, a quality-assurance manager, a citizen. Whether you are a school administrator, an architect, a newspaper editor, or an industry leader, you will recognize opportunities in every chapter. No doubt you will generate new strategies by virtue of your unique professional perspective. Turn the page; you are in for a treat.

Hershey, Pa. Mark D. Widome, M.D., M.P.H.
June 1990 Chair, Committee on Injury and Poison Prevention
American Academy of Pediatrics

PREFACE

This book is designed to encourage adults to make childhood injury prevention a high priority in their professional decisions. We have focused on childhood injury because children have special needs. Adults acknowledge a societal obligation to protect and guide children as an investment in the future. Because children lack judgment and experience, they cannot be expected to avoid injury on their own. It is unfair to blame them for injury which results from acting "childishly." Adults must grant children freedom from injury by providing a safe environment.

A developmental approach is useful in understanding the causes of injury and in planning prevention. The kinds of events in which a child is likely to be injured depend on the child's abilities and on where, how, and with whom the child spends time, all of which change as a child grows and matures. Children develop at different rates, and caretakers' decisions to grant independence are subjective, so age is only a crude correlate of developmental stage. In this book we categorize children as infants (up to 1 year of age), toddlers (1-2 years), preschoolers (3-5 years), elementary school ages (6-12 years), and young adolescents (13-15 years). Common injury risks within these categories are discussed. Individual children will pass through each of these stages, but not necessarily at the specified ages.

Some of the points, especially those focusing on the young adolescent, are relevant to older adolescents (16-19 years). Developmentally, older adolescents are in a unique period of transition. Their injury patterns come to resemble those of adults because they adopt increasingly adult behavior. They operate motorized vehicles, join the work force, and consume alcohol. Suicide occurs more frequently. Since we could not adequately address both their special needs and those of younger children in one volume, we have reluctantly limited our scope.

Chapter 1 presents the general facts about childhood injury. Chapter 2 introduces some of the opportunities for prevention that rest with each of nine different groups of adults. Detailed information about specific events leading to injury is presented in chapters 3 through 17, which are roughly grouped according to types of environments (e.g., The Roadway Environment; The Home Environment; The School and Recreational Environment). In each of these chapters, the facts relating to the designated injury topic are first summarized and then the developmental issues affecting the occurrence of injury and its prevention are discussed. Strategies for preventing such injuries are highlighted in boxed fashion and are subsequently presented at greater length in sections addressed to specific professional groups. The end of each chapter includes a list of additional reading material and resources.

We have not limited ourselves to what have often been termed "accidents" because life does not so limit children's experience. Unfortunately, along with an often needlessly high rate of unintentional injury for all children, there is a very real threat of deliberately inflicted injury for many. When one begins at the end point of injury, it is often impossible to determine the degree of culpability of adults responsible for the child. Uncertainty need not immobilize us. Many acts of intervention can become a part of the physical or social environment, thus protecting children from injury, no matter what the intent. We have focused on preventing injury rather than assigning blame. Comments concerning intentional injury are interspersed throughout our discussion whenever they seem appropriate to the injury topic. In addition to these scattered comments, chapter 13 is devoted to assault and chapter 14 to child suicide.

No type of childhood injury can be reduced substantially without the concerted action of many adult decision makers. Although we acknowledge that the duties of a given reader cannot always be correctly deduced from a professional title or work setting, for convenience we have addressed our suggestions to the following groups:

- schools and child care centers
- health care providers
- public agencies
- legislators and regulators
- law enforcement professionals
- voluntary organizations
- designers, architects, builders, and engineers
- business and industry
- mass media

It is quite possible that readers will find material of interest to them in one or more of these sections. Many adults have complex and multiple roles, and the categories are very broad and at times overlapping. Yet each group has something unique to offer to the field of injury prevention.

The hurried reader may find immediate guidance to the most pressing questions by consulting the facts section of a given chapter, as well as the section addressed to the appropriate professional role. At a more opportune moment, this basic understanding can be enhanced by a thorough perusal and by exploring the additional resources listed at the end of each chapter and in the appendix.

Baltimore, Md.   M. H. W., S. P. B., S. P. T., S. S., J. G.
Chicago, Il.
April 1990

ACKNOWLEDGMENTS

We would like to thank the Carnegie Corporation of New York for making childhood injury prevention one of its priorities and for the financial support and encouragement that made this book possible.

A book as broad in scope as this one could not be written without the help of professionals in many different fields. We are grateful for the interest and advice offered by the following people who served as advisors at the start of the project. Their comments have been useful in shaping the contents and organization of the book: Ms. Ardis Bell of the National Congress of Parents and Teachers (PTA); Mr. Milton Boyce of the 4-H program of the U.S. Department of Agriculture; Ms. Ellen Galinsky, formerly of the National Association for Education of Young Children and now of the Families and Work Institute; Dr. Joseph Greensher of the American Academy of Pediatrics; Mr. Christopher Gribbs of the American Institute of Architects; Dr. J. Alex Haller, Jr., of the American College of Surgeons; Dr. Stephen Hargarten of the American College of Emergency Physicians; Mr. Jerry Hershovitz of the Centers for Disease Control; Mr. Charles Hurley, formerly of the National Safety Council and now of the Insurance Institute for Highway Safety; Ms. Katherine McCarter of the American Public Health Association; Ms. Suzanne Randolph, formerly of the American Red Cross; Ms. Barbara Rawn of the National Committee for Prevention of Child Abuse; Ms. Joann Rodgers of the Office of Public Affairs of Johns Hopkins Medical Institutions; Ms. Carol L. Rogers of the American Association for the Advancement of Science; Mr. George W. Rutherford, Jr., of the Consumer Product Safety Commission; Ms. Betty Stewart of the Administration for Children, Youth, and Families; and Dr. Brian L. Wilcox of the American Psychological Association.

We enlisted the aid of some talented professionals to review book sections pertinent to their field and comment on our wording, to suggest additional references, and to answer specific questions. We are grateful for their unflagging attention to detail, their helpful suggestions, their willingness to help even after their initial job was done, and their general interest in the project. Captain Raymond D. Cotton, Northern Troop Commander, Maryland State Police, reviewed the sections for law enforcement professionals; Ms. Lisa Hillman, Director of Public Affairs, Johns Hopkins Children's Center, and Dr. Stewart M. Hoover, Associate Professor, School of Communications and Theater, Temple University, reviewed the sections for the mass media; Mr. Jake Pauls, Life Safety Specialist, Hughes Associates, Inc., of Wheaton, Maryland, reviewed the sections for designers, architects, builders, and engineers; and Mr. George W. Rutherford, Jr., Senior Epidemiologist, Consumer Product Safety Commission, reviewed the sections for legislators and regulators and for business and industry. We would also like to thank Dr. Andrew L. Dannenberg, Assistant Professor, Johns Hopkins Injury Prevention Center, Johns Hopkins School of Public Health, who reviewed chapter 6, Bicycles, and Dr. Garen J. Wintemute, Associate Professor, School of Medicine, University of California, Davis, who reviewed chapter 12, Firearms. The book was greatly improved by the advice of these consultants; it does not necessarily reflect their opinions or emphases, however, but rather our own. They should share the praise where we have succeeded but not the blame for any omissions or errors.

Experts exist who have detailed knowledge of the prevention strategies and resources available for a particular type of injury. In our efforts to compile a thorough resource for all types of childhood injury, we contacted many of these specialists, who always took time from their own work to answer our questions, to suggest references and resources, and to mail materials as needed. We are grateful to dozens of such individuals who helped to inform us before and as we wrote. We have chosen not to try to list all of you here, certain that we would make many omissions inadvertently.

We are grateful to our secretaries for their outstanding help. Finally, we owe a great debt to our families, especially the 13 children we are raising and have raised, who made daily sacrifices so that we could devote ourselves to the task of preventing injury to children, in which we share a vital interest.

CONTENTS

I INTRODUCTION

1 *The Injury Problem*   3
2 *The Role of Decision Makers*   14

II THE ROADWAY ENVIRONMENT

3 *Motor Vehicle Occupants*   29
4 *Users of Other Motor Vehicles*   46
5 *Pedestrians*   57
6 *Bicyclists*   68

III THE HOME ENVIRONMENT

7 *Fires and Burns*   85
8 *Poisoning*   100
9 *Choking and Suffocation*   111
10 *Falls*   127
11 *Animals*   140
12 *Firearms*   149
13 *Assaults*   161
14 *Suicide and Suicide Attempts*   172

IV THE SCHOOL AND RECREATION ENVIRONMENT

15 *Playground Injuries*   189

16 *Sports Injuries*   203

17 *Drowning and Other Water-Related Injuries*   217

CONCLUDING REMARKS: *A Call to Action*   231

APPENDIX: *Selected Sources of General Information About Childhood Injury Prevention*   233

INDEX   237

I
INTRODUCTION

1
The Injury Problem

Injuries are the leading childhood health problem in the United States (see figure 1-1). Each year about 10,000 children under the age of 15 die from injury (see figure 1-2). Many of them die immediately, before any rescue unit can arrive to begin the process of emergency care. Since fatal injuries often strike the young, more years of productive life are lost to injury than to any disease. This is a national tragedy. Preventing these injuries should be a compelling concern.

Deaths are only part of the problem. For every death, 34 children are admitted to a hospital for the treatment of injury. And for every injured child admitted to a hospital, 30 more are treated in an emergency department. Each year, about one out of every five children in this country suffers an injury for which medical care is sought (Gallagher et al. 1984). Too often, there are lasting effects. Injuries may result in disability or disfigurement, impairing the child's development, future well-being, and achievements.

As public health measures and improvements in the standard of living have markedly reduced the impact of common childhood infectious diseases, the injury problem has become increasingly prominent. Although in recent years the number of childhood injury deaths has decreased modestly, much more could be achieved by the concentrated and cooperative effort of the many people whose decisions affect children.

Patterns of Childhood Injury

For almost every kind of injury at every age after infancy, males are at higher risk than females (Rivara et al. 1982). Male death rates are only slightly higher than rates for females for motor vehicle–occupant deaths prior to adolescence, for example, but nearly five times as many male children as female become unintentional firearm fatalities (Baker and Waller 1989). The factors that lead to this increased risk for males are complex and difficult to untangle. They may include inborn differences in behavior as well as obvious differences in exposure related to traditional male and

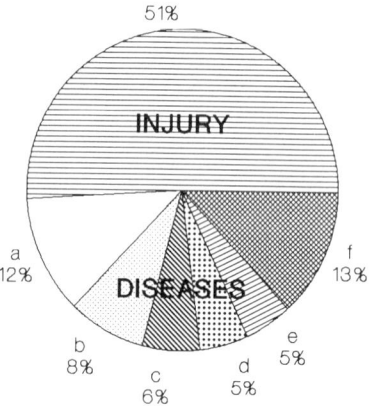

FIGURE 1-1. *Proportion of childhood deaths from injury compared with other causes, ages 1-14, U.S., 1986. Key: (a) neoplasms (cancer); (b) congenital anomalies; (c) diseases of the nervous system and sense organs; (d) diseases of the circulatory system; (e) diseases of the respiratory system; (f) all others. (Source: National Center for Health Statistics 1988.)*

female roles in our society. Subtle differences in socialization operating at a very early age may produce gender-dependent differences in risk taking.

Injuries vary not only by age and sex but by geography. Analysis of childhood injury deaths for the six years from 1980 through 1985 revealed wide disparities in death rates among states (Waller et al. 1989). A threefold difference was found between the state with the highest rate (Alaska) and the state with the lowest (Massachusetts). Southern and mountain states tended to have high rates; the New England, Middle Atlantic, and midwestern states had lower rates. Distinct geographical patterns were also revealed by mapping rates for particular events. For instance, motor vehicle–occupant deaths were found to be particularly high in the South and Southwest, drowning deaths in the Pacific Coast and Gulf states, house-fire deaths in the Southeast, unintentional firearm deaths in the South, and suicide in the northern and mountain states.

Within any broad geographical area there appear to be marked differences which depend not only on whether a child lives on a farm or in the city, for instance, but also on socioeconomic status. Poor children are much more likely to die from injury than are children of families with more economic resources. Children in low-income areas more often experience certain injury events (like house fire or assault) which are often fatal. A large proportion of the difference in injury rates often noted among races is probably accounted for by differences in socioeconomic status.

Injuries also vary by intent. There is little doubt that many intentionally inflicted injuries are mislabeled "accidents." Though it is highly desirable to identify abused children and to help troubled families, it will never be possible to cleanly separate all injuries into categories by intent. The blurring of distinctions between unintentional ("accidental") injury, injury resulting from neglect, and intentional injury is seen when the range of responsibility for injury, or "spectrum of intent," is explored even briefly (Garbarino 1988).

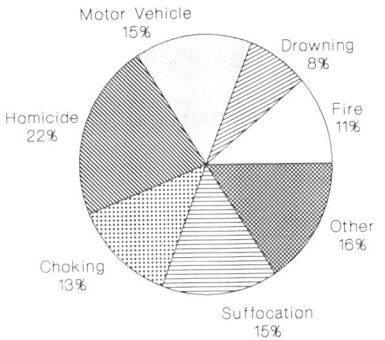
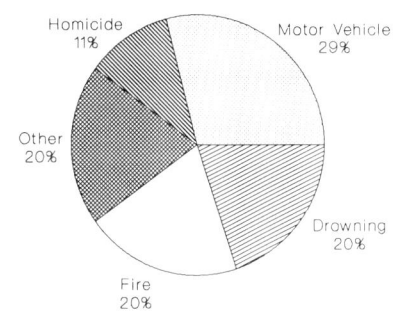
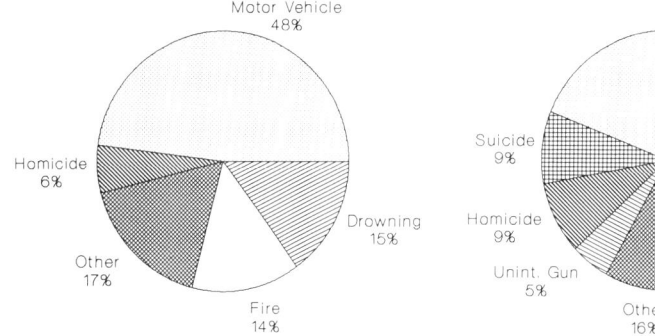

FIGURE 1-2. *Injury deaths in U.S. children by cause, 1986. Numbers in wedges represent percentage of total in each age-group. (Source: National Center for Health Statistics 1988.)*

Spectrum of Intent

Traditionally, unintentional injury events have been called "accidents," a term that suggests the harm could not have been reasonably prevented. When a knowledge base develops which allows an informed parent or other decision maker to anticipate and thus reduce the likelihood of a particular injury event, society redefines resulting injuries as "preventable." Attempts are made to educate adults and children about preventable events and to decrease risk through environmental controls and community services. A salient example is the ingestion of toxic substances by exploring toddlers: parents are warned by their health care providers, regulations require child-resistant packaging, and poison-control centers provide postingestion advice. Gradually, society comes to expect responsible adults to recognize and prevent such events.

When adults, products, or environments fail to meet the community's expectations for minimal standards of care, resulting injuries are said to have resulted from neglect and negligence (Garbarino 1988). Manufacturers, builders, organizations, and other responsible parties may be sued. Children may be removed from the homes of neglectful parents. Gradually, the definition of neglect changes. Motor vehicle–occupant injuries were once assumed to be unpreventable. As knowledge about the value of seat belts and car safety seats grew, these injuries became "preventable." Now the parent of a young child injured in a crash while sitting on the parent's lap may be considered neglectful. At the far end of the spectrum of intent are attacks and assaults inflicted upon children. Child abuse and self-inflicted injuries are in this category.

Categorization of injury by intent is blurred not only by progress in the art and science of prevention but also by issues of ethics, policy, and psychology. Some assaults on children, specifically those labeled corporal punishment, are widely practiced and condoned. Some adults see injury as necessary for learning. Further, in some situations, intent to harm is unconscious or submerged. Stressed or angry parents may not recognize their own motivation for failing to break the chain of events that leads to injury.

Fortunately, at any point along the spectrum of intent, many prevention strategies provide protection. Many can do so without requiring individual acts by parents or children. If water heaters do not produce water hot enough to scald skin, tap-water burns can be avoided whether the caregiver is ignorant of the danger, neglectful, or deliberately douses the child in a moment of misguided disciplinary action or rage.

Targeting Prevention Efforts

Looking at the broad strokes which describe injury risk—age, sex, geography, socioeconomic status, intent—one might conclude that the injury problem can be cured by focusing on small, high-risk segments of the population. It is true that injury-prevention efforts need to be targeted, but every child is at risk. Prevention efforts need to be tailored to the particular injury events most likely to occur, but all children need attention. Injury is a widespread disease. Like immunizations, all children need injury prevention. All need the standard package; some need even more.

Within groups of the same age, sex, geographical locale, and socioeconomic status, investigators have long been interested in predicting which individuals are most likely to be injured because of some innate characteristic—that is, those who are "accident-prone." Many observers of children believe in the concept of accident-proneness, but it has not been confirmed by careful research (Langley 1982). Certainly, there are some children who are injured repeatedly, but injuries are common enough that this may be due most often to chance alone or to environmental and social factors. To predict which individual of the many who are at risk will actually be injured is not possible with our current level of knowledge. Our preventive measures must be designed to protect all.

Though it is not often possible to predict which particular child will be injured, injuries among a population are predictable events that can and should be prevented. If a bicycling child not wearing a helmet rides out of a driveway into the path of an oncoming car, it is misleading to refer to the resulting head injury as an "accident." It was really quite predictable.

Concepts of Injury Prevention

Webster's defines the word *accident* as "an event which takes place without one's foresight or expectation; an event which proceeds from an unknown cause, or is an unusual effect of a known cause and therefore was not expected." Learning to foresee "accidents" is the first step in preventing them, and it is the second definition of accident—"an unfortunate occurrence or mishap, especially one resulting in an injury"—which provides the appropriate focus on the outcome of the accident: the injury. The injury can often be prevented, even if the mishap was not. A clear example is the car seat belt. Seat belts do not prevent highway crashes. They do, however, reduce the likelihood of injury should a crash occur.

Most injuries are caused by mechanical energy (the energy of motion) impinging on the body. Some are caused by thermal or chemical energy. In the terminology used by epidemiologists working to eliminate infectious diseases, energy is the "agent" which can cause the "disease" (injury) in a susceptible "host" (a person) (Haddon 1980). The disease results when the agent and the host interact in an environment which permits it. We can prevent injuries by preventing these interactions or by providing a way to discharge the energy without harming the body. For example, restraining a child in a car safety seat allows energy to dissipate safely in the event of a car crash as the child slows down with the car rather than being flung against its interior.

Strategies to prevent injuries can be directed toward preventing events which might cause injury (pre-event-phase strategies); or toward protecting individuals against injury should a mishap occur (event-phase strategies); or toward minimizing the consequences after an injury through prompt and skilled emergency services, medical care, and rehabilitation designed to deal with the special needs of the injured child (post-event-phase strategies). Strategies from all three phases are important in controlling each type of injury (see table 1-1).

Table 1-1. Injury Control Strategies, by Relationship to Event

Relationship to Event	Purpose of Strategies	Examples: Drowning	Examples: Intentional Self-poisoning
Pre-event phase	To prevent events which might cause injury	Four-sided fencing for pools	Diagnosing and treating depression
Event phase	To prevent injury when event occurs	Personal flotation devices	Limiting total amount of medication prescribed
Post-event phase	To prevent unnecessary severity or disability when an injury has occurred	Cardiopulmonary resuscitation	Removing toxic substance from the body by lavage or dialysis

Probably the most common injury-prevention strategy employed by and recommended to parents is that they "watch" their children and keep them "out of danger." No doubt parental supervision has prevented and will continue to prevent many injurious mishaps. In fact, considering the many hazards with which a child must cope, one might be amazed that there are not even more injuries. Often parents are working at the top of their personal capacity to protect their children from injury. Parents can never be made aware of all the injury risks their children face, nor can they supervise their children every minute. Parents need the help of the many others whose decisions can reduce the risk of injury for their children—legislators, regulators, health professionals, teachers and school administrators, day care providers, lawyers, law enforcement officers, fire fighters, voluntary service groups, community workers, social workers, philanthropists, designers, architects, reporters, producers and directors, manufacturers, and the business community. If all responsible adults attend to the task of preventing injury to children in their professional decisions, protection can be built into the environment and into the way society operates. The result will be children who are free from injury without requiring from their parents encyclopedic knowledge, unlimited resources, unyielding vigilance, and constant control of the child's behavior.

Strategies which protect on every occasion without the action of the parent or child are called "passive" or automatic. Marketing children's aspirin in small bottles which contain nonlethal amounts is an example of automatic protection assured by those who manufacture medications. At the opposite end of the spectrum are strategies that require action by individuals every time protection is needed. Storing toxic substances away from toddlers is an example. Such efforts are very troublesome and leave many opportunities for failure. Consistent use by most of the population is rarely achieved.

Some strategies are partially automatic—they require some action by individuals. Strategies which are not fully automatic can be very effective when used, as is the case with child-resistant caps for medications. However, the potential for misuse leading to inadequate protection is often high, as in the following examples: adults may request that their own medication be supplied without the special caps, for ease of opening; users may leave the caps off; children may learn to open them. In general, when effective automatic strategies are available they are more attractive than those requiring frequent individual action because they offer the most comprehensive protection with the least bother (Baker 1981) (see figure 1-3).

Implementation of Prevention Strategies

A number of approaches are available for encouraging the use of injury-prevention strategies. Education must go beyond simple transfer of information. It must motivate change. Education of decision makers is crucial. Key figures in many different professional roles must see the need to provide protection for children. Though this is a challenging task, it is not as formidable as setting out to educate all parents and children about all necessary injury-prevention strategies and making sure they invariably comply. The decisions of people in powerful positions can add incentives or remove barriers to injury prevention (Baker 1981). For example, insurance companies might lower the cost of home insurance for homes with automatic sprinkler systems. Community groups and health-related agencies

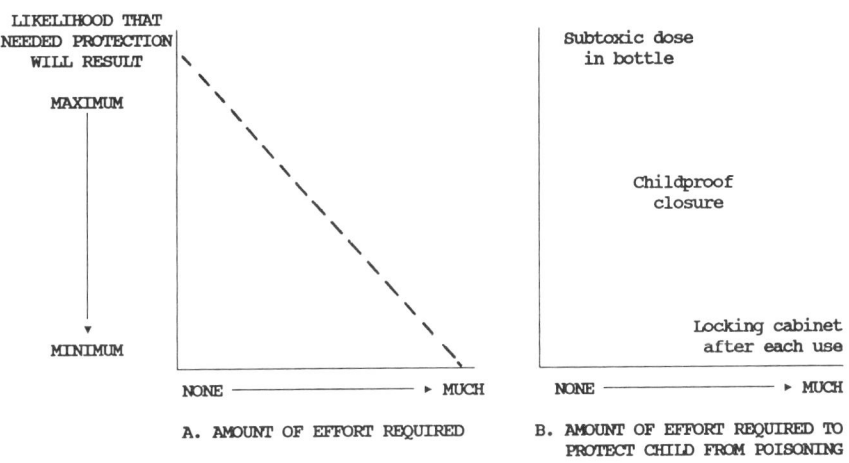

FIGURE 1-3. *Relationship between the amount of effort required in order for a child to be protected and the likelihood that the protection will, in fact, result. A. In general; B. With examples pertinent to poisoning. (From Baker 1981. Copyright 1981 by* Journal of Public Health Policy. *Reprinted by permission.)*

can establish rental programs to make car safety seats more convenient to obtain and less costly.

Educated and motivated decision makers can make use of a number of proven approaches. Environmental modification, design changes, legislation, regulation, and litigation have all been used successfully to prevent childhood injuries. Most often a number of approaches must be used together. For example, the multifaceted "Children Can't Fly" program, begun in the Bronx, New York, in 1972 to reduce children's falls from windows, combined voluntary reporting of falls, door-to-door community outreach, a public awareness campaign through the media, and distribution of free, easy-to-install window guards. Window-fall fatalities decreased in the city and particularly in the Bronx. Subsequently, the New York City Health Code was amended to require owners of multiple-family dwellings to provide window guards in apartments housing children. The amendment was upheld on challenge in the state's courts (Spiegel and Lindaman 1977).

Legislation for safety is most often created at the state level, such as laws now existing in every state requiring the use of specially designed car seats for young children (Teret et al. 1986). Regulations are created by administrative bodies or agencies, often at the federal level, to ensure the safety of products sold in interstate commerce. An example is the Consumer Product Safety Commission (CPSC) regulation that governs the design of cribs (Federal Hazardous Substances Act 1988).

Litigation has been useful when education, legislation, and regulation have failed to address safety problems. For example, transferring the cost of injuries back to the manufacturer of an unsafe product gives a strong incentive for product improvement. The design of some unsafe hot-water vaporizers was changed after successful lawsuits were brought by burned children against the manufacturer (Teret 1981).

Sometimes objections are made to strategies that go beyond education on the grounds that they interfere with personal freedom. Environmental modifications actually provide more freedom for a child to grow, develop, and explore without restrictions. Legislation requiring the use of safety equipment like seat belts, car safety seats, or helmets can be seen as a necessary step to widespread public acceptance of these measures which will permit children to reach adulthood free from the ravages of injury. There are many precedents for society's providing children with at least a minimal standard of care, such as food, immunizations, and schooling. Protection from injury should be added to the list. It is a wise investment.

Challenge to Decision Makers

To reduce the toll from injury during childhood, adults who make the decisions which affect children must use the full range of injury-prevention approaches to avoid the creation of new injury hazards, eliminate or modify existing hazards, put into place strategies that are known to work and are as automatic as practical, encourage the use of injury-prevention strategies by adding incentives or eliminating barriers, and assure adequate emergency and rehabilitative care for injured children (Wilson and Baker 1987). Leadership is needed in many arenas. Chapter 2 addresses the specific opportunities and obligations for reducing childhood injury which are an integral part of adult decision-making roles.

References

Baker, SP. 1981. Childhood injuries: The community approach to prevention. *J Public Health Policy* 2(3):235-246.
Baker, SP, and Waller, AE. 1989. *Childhood Injury: State-by-State Mortality Facts*. Baltimore, Md.: Johns Hopkins University Injury Prevention Center.
Consumer Product Safety Commission. 1988. Requirements for full-size baby cribs. 16 *CFR* 1508.
Gallagher, SS, et al. 1984. The incidence of injuries among 87,000 Massachusetts children and adolescents: Results of the 1980-81 Statewide Childhood Injury Prevention Program surveillance system. *Am J Public Health* 74:1340-1347.
Garbarino, J. 1988. Preventing childhood injury: Developmental and mental health issues. *Am J Orthopsychiatry* 58(1):25-45.
Haddon, W Jr. 1980. Advances in the epidemiology of injuries as a basis for public policy (Landmarks in American Epidemiology). *Public Health Rep* 95(5): 411-421.
Langley, J. 1982. The "accident prone" child—the perpetration of a myth. *Aust Paediatr J* 18:243-246.
National Center for Health Statistics. 1988. *Vital Statistics of the United States, 1986*. Vol. 2, Mortality, pt. A. Dept. of Health and Human Services Publication No. (PHS) 88-1122. Washington, D.C.: U.S. Government Printing Office.
Rivara, FP, et al. 1982. Epidemiology of childhood injuries: II. Sex differences in injury rates. *Am J Dis Child* 136:502-506.
Spiegel, CN, and Lindaman, FC. 1977. Children can't fly: A program to prevent childhood morbidity and mortality from window falls. *Am J Public Health* 67(12):1143-1147.
Teret, S. 1981. Injury control and product liability. *J Public Health Policy* 2(1): 4957.
Teret, SP, et al. 1986. Child restraint laws: An analysis of gaps in coverage. *Am J Public Health* 76(1):31-34.
Waller, AE, et al. 1989. Childhood injury deaths: National analysis and geographic variations. *Am J Public Health* 79(3):310-315.
Wilson, MH, and Baker, SP. 1987. Structural approach to injury control. *Journal of Social Issues* 43:73-86.

Additional Sources of Information

Alpert, J, and Guyer, B (eds.). 1985. Symposium on Injuries and Injury Prevention. *Pediatr Clin North Am* 32(1).
American Academy of Pediatrics. 1987. *Injury Control for Children and Youth*. Elk Grove Village, Ill.: American Academy of Pediatrics.

Baker, SP, et al. In press. *The Injury Fact Book*, ed. 2. New York: Oxford University Press.
Baker, SP, et al. 1984. *The Injury Fact Book.* Lexington, Mass.: Lexington Books.
Berger, LR. 1981. Childhood injuries: Recognition and prevention. *Curr Probl Pediatr* 12(1):1–59.
Bergman, AB (ed.). 1982. *Preventing Childhood Injuries.* Columbus, Ohio: Ross Laboratories.
Christoffel, T. 1989. Injury Prevention, special issue. *Law, Medicine and Health Care* 17(1).
Ciccheti, D. 1989. *Child Maltreatment: Theory and Research on the Causes and Consequences of Child Abuse and Neglect.* New York: Cambridge University Press.
Committee on Trauma Research. 1985. *Injury in America: A Continuing Public Health Problem.* Washington, D.C.: National Academy Press.
Garbarino, J, and Gilliam, G. 1980. *Understanding Abusive Families.* Lexington, Mass.: Lexington Books.
Guyer, B, et al. 1989. Prevention of childhood injuries: Evaluation of the Statewide Childhood Injury Prevention Program (SCIPP). *Am J Public Health* 79(11):1521–1527.
Haddon, W Jr, and Baker, SP. 1981. Injury control, in Clark, D, and MacMahon, B (eds.): *Preventive and Community Medicine.* Boston: Little Brown, pp. 109–140.
Harrington, C, et al. 1988. *Injury Prevention Programs in State Health Departments: A National Survey.* Report of the Childhood Injury Prevention Resource Center. Boston: Harvard School of Public Health.
Kane, DN. 1985. *Environmental Hazards to Young Children.* Phoenix: Oryx Press.
Kempe, CH, and Helfer, RE (eds.). 1987. *The Battered Child*, ed. 4. Chicago: University of Chicago Press.
Kraus, JF, et al. 1986. Incidence, severity, and external causes of pediatric brain injury. *Am J Dis Child* 140(7):687–693.
National Academy of Sciences. 1988. *Injury Control.* Washington, D.C.: National Academy Press.
National Committee for Injury Prevention and Control. 1989. *Injury Prevention: Meeting the Challenge.* New York: Oxford University Press.
National Safety Council. 1988. *Accident Facts.* Chicago: National Safety Council.
Pless, IB, and Arsenault, L. 1987. The role of health education in the prevention of injuries to children. *Journal of Social Issues* 43(2):87–103.
Rice, DP, et al. 1989. *Cost of Injury in the United States: A Report to Congress 1989.* San Francisco: Institute for Health and Aging, University of California and Injury Prevention Center, The Johns Hopkins University.
Rivara, FP. 1982. Epidemiology of childhood injuries: I. Review of current research and presentation of conceptual framework. *Am J Dis Child* 136:399–405.
Rivara, FP, et al. 1989. Population-based study of unintentional injury incidence and impact during childhood. *Am J Public Health* 79:990–994.
Roberts, MC, and Brooks, PH (eds.). 1987. Children's injuries: Prevention and public policy. *Journal of Social Issues* (special issue) 43(2).
Robertson, LS. 1983. *Injuries: Causes, Control Strategies, and Public Policy.* Lexington, Mass.: Lexington Books.

Runyan, CW, and Gerken, EA. 1989. Epidemiology and prevention of adolescent injury: A review and research agenda. *JAMA* 262(16):2273-2279.

Waller, JA. 1985. *Injury Control: A Guide to the Causes and Prevention of Trauma*. Lexington, Mass.: Lexington Books.

Wissow, LS. 1990. *Child Advocacy for the Clinician: An Approach to Child Abuse and Neglect*. Baltimore: Williams and Wilkins.

2
The Role of Decision Makers

It is hard to imagine an adult who does not, in a professional or public role, bear some responsibility for preventing injury for populations of children as well as for the children in his or her own family. Adults design, manufacture, market, and sell the vehicles children ride on and in. They design, surface, and police the roads on which they ride. Adults build the buildings in which children learn, play, and live. They decide whether there will be a sprinkler system to put out fires. Adults decide whether the pool will be fenced and a railing put up at the dock. They determine whether private use of fireworks will be legal and how high to heat water. Adults decide whether to require a waiting period before handguns are purchased and whether to report injuries to agencies charged with protecting children from being battered by their parents. Adults decide who will drive the school bus and how new it will be, whether a parent will take four or eight children in a private car on the school trip to the zoo, what surfacing will be under the slide, and whether seat belts will be discussed in health class. Adults decide whether the catcher has to wear a face mask and whether the dizzy football player goes back into the game. They decide whether to devote column inches to the protective value of bicycle helmets and whether to show the television hero wearing a seat belt. Adults decide whether children will sleep in pajamas that are flame-retardant and which toy will be given away free with a child's hamburger.

As such a list is expanded and made more specific, it becomes clear that most adults can be injury-prevention specialists. Few adults, if any, wish to cause injuries to children, and most would say preventing injuries is important to them. Most adults have unique opportunities to do so within their professional and community leadership roles. The remainder of this chapter outlines broadly the injury-control challenges and strategies integral to a number of professional settings and decision-making roles.

2.A Schools and Child Care Centers

Schools and child care centers are in a particularly advantageous position to advocate and practice injury prevention. In their traditional, instructional role, educators can present injury-prevention information in the classroom, as a separate unit or incorporated with other subjects, directed to the students' developmental age and to activities popular in that particular locale and at that grade level. "Safety education" can also be presented as organized extracurricular activities—for example, a trip to the science museum to see how air bags work. If school-age children become better at injury prevention, other children may benefit indirectly—specifically, younger siblings or other children for whom schoolchildren baby-sit and their own children when they have them.

Schools and child care center personnel are in a prime position to enlist support from other members of the community, such as law enforcement and fire department personnel, members of voluntary service organizations, or health professionals. Schools can also involve parents by recruiting them to aid in injury-prevention activities, offering special parent-education workshops geared to specific injury problems, sending home companion materials to accompany students' lessons, or encouraging injury-prevention initiatives by parent-teacher organizations.

Because parents entrust children to their care, schools and child care centers should scrupulously practice injury prevention. They are permitted, even expected, to insist on reasonable behavioral protocols and thus can regulate potentially hazardous activities on school grounds, such as bike riding or skateboarding. Even more importantly, schools are expected to make their own environments safe for children and should make modifications as necessary; these can serve as an example for children, parents, and visitors. Schools' guidance should extend to educating parents and children about safe travel to and from school. School systems have a special obligation to assure safe equipment, operation, and behavior for school busing and other school-sponsored activities.

Schools must play a key role in identifying and protecting children who may be showing signs of abuse or neglect. No other institution may interact regularly with such children. School personnel should be trained to recognize and report suspicious injuries or behavior patterns and to work with the appropriate agencies to protect children when indicated.

Schools and child care facilities should institute reporting procedures for injuries occurring on school grounds. Data should be reviewed regularly to identify the major hazards and circumstances of injury and should be shared with appropriate individuals or groups, within the school or without, who are responsible for instituting protective measures or policymaking. Special attention should be given to collecting data on after-school injuries, especially those related to interscholastic and informal sports; these constitute the largest number of serious injuries occurring in connection with school yet often go uncounted because they occur after hours or off school property.

Finally, since the children of today are the decision makers of tomorrow, schools should provide curricula that will enable children to consider the design of environments and products as well as policies and prejudices that influence injury risks. The science of injury prevention can be taught in a variety of contexts ranging from the physics of motion to the characteristics of various animals — and may be better received than anything labeled "safety education." Civics classes are an ideal setting in which children can learn about influencing legislators or the media. One group of schoolchildren, for example, persuaded a television hero to wear his seat belt whenever he's shown in a motor vehicle. Schoolchildren in another locale, worried about the serious head injuries classmates sustained while biking, stimulated adults to draft, debate, and pass an innovative helmet law for their county.

2.B Health Care Providers

The role of the provider of pediatric health services in injury prevention is pivotal since health care providers (along with health researchers) are in a position to recognize the dimensions of injury problems and detect new patterns and associations as well as to inform patients, parents, the public, and decision makers. Since health care providers must deal directly with consequences of injury for many children, an active interest in injury prevention is their right, if not even their obligation. However, the role must be defined much more broadly than it usually is.

Health professionals must prevent childhood injury at their own offices, clinics, and hospital practice sites. In these locations even the most basic prevention strategies are often ignored. Babies are dressed on high surfaces from which they may fall, hospital cribs may have overly wide slat spacing through which tiny bodies may slip, nurses may quiet fretful infants with makeshift pacifiers which can pull apart and choke the sucking child, poisonous substances may be within reach of small hands, and few unused electrical outlets are covered. In addition to the direct effect on injury and liability risk, these practices present a poor model for parents to emulate.

Though physician advice to parents on safety or "accident prevention" is not new (Buchen 1800 quoted in Nader 1985), attention to injury prevention has gained momentum only recently (Pless and Arsenault 1987). Patient education on some injury issues is now considered routine, a part of standard practice (AAP 1988). Even so, there should be little expectation — and there is little evidence — that patient "education" as it is usually performed will produce behavioral change. Health care providers are rarely skilled in educational techniques and have little time and many disparate injury topics to cover. Injury prevention will be only one item on the counseling agenda for a visit, taking its place among illness, nutritional, developmental, and behavioral issues to which both the parent and the health professional may give higher priority. Counseling on injury prevention may increase the patient's or parent's perception of injury risk and may add to their knowledge, but even these successes do not lead reliably to behavioral change, the likelihood of which will be affected by many additional factors the physician has rarely explored or affected.

Certainly, patient education is more likely to precipitate behavioral change when it is built on sound educational theory. Such educational efforts take additional time, energy, skills, and resources and must be targeted to the appropriate risk group and a limited number of strategies. Even perfect patient education could not be expected to solve the childhood injury problem because not all children are regularly seen by health care providers and those who are have less frequent contacts as they age. Recommended health supervision visits for young children are timed to coincide with an adequate immunization schedule and may not pace injury-prevention counseling appropriately. Even given these difficulties, very young children and their parents are seen by the health professionals more reliably perhaps than in any other institution, so health care providers have a unique opportunity to influence behavioral patterns. Health professionals are also allowed by families to advise them on the most intimate details of their behavior and family life, so injury topics are not "off-limits." The fact that patient education cannot stand alone as the solitary injury-prevention strategy does not mean that health care providers should abandon it but that they must improve upon it by becoming better at it and must enhance it with other strategies. Education can build the climate of awareness in which other strategies are accepted.

Health care providers must not limit their activities to their offices and to individual patient encounters, however, or their pediatric patients will be poorly served. Physicians have often led the campaign for effective public strategies to prevent childhood injury. One public health pediatrician was responsible for the nation's first car safety seat law, for example, and physicians have led the way to poisoning-prevention measures and to control of tap-water scalds. When health professionals speak knowledgeably and with the interests of children obviously on their lips, other decision makers listen. The health professional's role in preventing injury includes writing letters, speaking to groups of children and parents, advising about safety in day care and schools, serving as a team physician who emphasizes prevention as well as treatment, calling the Consumer Product Safety Commission to report a product-related injury, testifying before legislatures, reporting cases of suspected abuse, intervening in cases of family dysfunction which may lead to injury, and voting. Childhood's biggest health problem deserves no less from those who have accepted responsibility for children's health.

2.C Public Agencies

Although agencies may not define their role in injury-prevention terms, the activities of many impact on the occurrence of injury because public agencies are charged with enforcing policies and procedures and maintaining environments. Standards for day care homes and centers, residential buildings, public buildings, roadways, and recreational areas and activities are examples. Once established, codes and regulations should be enforced through inspections or other activities and reviewed regularly.

Agencies also control the quality, and often the use, of important injury-related data. Health departments have access to injury mortality data for the state, and many also have registries of hospital-discharge data. Providing good data for agencies and groups to use as a basis for program decisions is a crucial role of health departments. Detailed mortality data on childhood injuries are available for 1980–1985 (Baker and Waller 1989); states can update these data and subdivide by county in order to provide local data. Other agencies can be active in collecting and analyzing injury data, for example on fires or motor vehicle crashes. Reporting systems should be designed to be interactive with those in other states (see section 2.D).

State and local health agencies can serve as the leads to coordinate regional injury-control activities and to build coalitions of organizations, groups, and individuals working for injury prevention. Resources are available to help establish injury-prevention programs either as separate entities or working within existing frameworks and to train public and private health personnel to implement childhood injury–prevention initiatives in their programs, clinics, and communities (Micik et al. 1987). The nature of injury prevention calls for a multidisciplinary approach, so representatives from many different agencies must work in concert. An excellent resource for agencies working in injury prevention is the book *Injury Prevention: Meeting the Challenge* (National Committee for Injury Prevention and Control 1989), which details how to organize a coalition, identify a problem, work with data, and design, implement, and evaluate a program. Evaluation is an integral part of any injury-prevention program. Agencies that cannot fund an adequate evaluation component can implement interventions that others have shown to be effective.

Singled out for particular mention are protective-service agencies, not only because of their acknowledged responsibility to respond to intentional injuries, but also because of their opportunities to prevent injury. Many protective-service agencies are limited by mandate, training, or resources to being "allegation driven" — that is, responding to reports of child maltreatment. If personnel cannot validate a specific allegation of harm or severe risk, they may be forced to end their involvement with a family. To become more effective in injury prevention, protective-service agencies must also focus on preventive services that assess the overall character of the child's family, environment, and community life and the degree to which these factors pose a risk to the child's well-being. Effective interventions need to be made available to protect children at risk. Protective-service agencies should require foster care providers to maintain high safety standards inside and outside the home; periodic checks should be made. Agency personnel should be willing and able to provide injury-prevention information in a nonpunitive fashion to help parents with the difficult job of guarding their children's safety. Educational home safety inspections for families with small children can be conducted by protective-service agency personnel in cooperation with personnel from other agencies with access to homes.

2.D Legislators and Regulators

Among the most effective tools for injury prevention are legislation and regulation. Well-designed evaluative studies have proven the ability of the law to reduce the incidence of injury; this is particularly true when the laws and rules are vigorously enforced. Laws that are restricted to secondary enforcement — where the violator can only be apprehended or penalized if he or she is caught violating another law — are less effective than laws subject to primary enforcement. Likewise, reliance on voluntary compliance with regulation is ineffective.

Legislators and regulators interested in injury data upon which to base laws and rules should contact academically based injury-prevention centers. These centers may also be helpful in creating model bills, providing expert testimony in legislative and administrative hearings, and evaluating the effect of laws.

Local lawmakers (e.g., members of city councils) should be aware of the long history of public health laws made at a local level. Examples include local ordinances which strictly prohibit private use of fireworks or the sale, purchase, or firing of firearms. In many states, home-rule provisions permit local lawmakers to address local issues regarding safety. Preemptive efforts of the federal and state governments should be opposed if they compromise safety in favor of vested business interests.

In general, state legislatures are given the power to protect the health and safety of the public. Although injury-prevention laws (e.g., motorcycle helmet laws) are sometimes opposed by groups asserting the importance of individuals' freedoms, legislation designed to protect childhood safety is often spared that battle because the state is expected to act paternalistically toward children who are unable to protect themselves.

Sometimes new legislation or regulatory changes are needed to enable effective data collecting, injury reporting, and tracking systems. This is important in the area of intentional injuries, for instance, where detecting repeat injuries is a high priority, and families may move across local and state boundaries and thus avoid detection by geographically limited data-collection systems.

Legislators and lobbyists interested in a particular form of injury prevention would be wise to cooperate with those supporting other injury bills in order to build a coalition of support for their goals. For example, as a result of a bicycling club's support of several bills to reduce drunk driving, Mothers Against Drunk Driving, a powerful highway safety lobby, offered to support future bicycle safety legislation (Baltimore Bicycling Club 1986).

2.E Law Enforcement Professionals

Strict enforcement of laws, even those promulgated with educational rather than punitive intent — for example, those requiring the use of safety seats and seat belts — will reduce injury. Law enforcement professionals can participate with other agencies and individuals in state or local coalitions to promote injury prevention through enforcement efforts, school programs, and public-education campaigns. Officers can work with other professional organizations for passage of injury-prevention legislation. Police have often been very effective witnesses in testifying before state legislatures — for example, to advocate child-restraint laws.

Too often, the function of law enforcement is seen as only investigatory and accusatory, after the commission of a wrongful act. The important role law enforcement officers (police, sheriffs, natural resource department personnel, fish and game patrols, special police, etc.) play in primary prevention of injuries often is given inadequate attention. Preventive action by law enforcement can take the form of assisting those at risk for injury, deterring harmful acts, and providing invaluable data through police reports upon which prevention strategies can be based.

Police can be trained to look for, recognize, and report to protective-service agencies any injuries related to child abuse or neglect. Police often play an important role in the investigations of these agencies.

Law enforcement departments can emphasize injury prevention among their own personnel and in their own facilities. Law enforcement officers are strong role models; they can protect themselves and influence others by wearing seat belts in cars, using and storing firearms correctly, and using personal flotation devices (PFDs) in boats, for example. Youth correctional facilities should be designed to protect the youths from both unintentional injuries (e.g., fires and burns) and intentional injuries (e.g., suicide).

People in law enforcement can help prevent childhood injuries by accurately recording data to be used in assessing possible sources of injury, trends, and affected populations. Data should not be limited to those which allocate human fault and should be determined in cooperation with a coalition of injury-prevention professionals to avoid gaps and to ensure that the data collected are as useful as possible. Reporting systems should be interactive with those in other jurisdictions (see Section 2.D, Legislators and Regulators).

2.F Voluntary Organizations

Groups already organized at the community level can be uniquely effective in injury-prevention efforts for many reasons. Churches, chambers of commerce, service clubs, recreational leagues, youth groups, social clubs — these are the fabric of the community, and their members make things work. While reflecting community mores, they also contain within their ranks the community leaders and the organizational structure to promote change.

Many of these groups deal directly with children and families and/or seek projects to promote community welfare. They are wise about what will work best in their community; they know the local barriers which must be overcome and the most effective incentives. Through their membership, their communications, their reputations, and their programs, they reach large proportions of the individuals in the community.

If voluntary organizations sponsor programs for children, they have the responsibility to provide protection from injury. Some examples are blatant. If children are transported in automobiles or vans, they should be properly restrained. Protective equipment and trained adult supervisors who make safety a priority are important for all sporting events. Facilities should be well designed and maintained. Such efforts not only reduce the likelihood of injury, the primary goal, but also reduce liability, a propitious side benefit for the organization.

Community groups can direct a special program toward decreasing a particular type of injury in their locale. They might offer car seat rental programs. They might adopt a playground and renovate it with injury prevention, as well as more creative use, as a goal. They might train members to provide hazard inspections and counseling in the homes of families with small children. They might organize a bicycle helmet campaign with the objective of reaching every child bicyclist in the community. They might raise money to fence an abandoned landfill or pressure the city council or state legislature to stiffen safety requirements for day care homes. They might provide conflict-resolution training for young adolescents. Many such examples will be given throughout the remainder of this book. Consulting with experts will help communities to expend resources on strategies most likely to work. Evaluation is highly desirable.

Community organizations are the necessary partners in any coalition which addresses the unique problems of childhood injury on a local level. The diverse injury events which may befall children in their daily lives require cooperative effort. Priority problems and opportunities to act will differ from community to community. An arrangement in which health care providers, local governmental agencies, schools, and community organizations work together toward a common goal is ideal, since each of these groups has an intimate role in the lives of the children who live in the community. The adults who fill these roles serve as parental surrogates, but none more so than the members of organizations who represent the responsible adults—the people in charge—in a community. If they are not looking after the health of their children, who will?

2.G Designers, Architects, Builders, and Engineers

Quite simply stated, most severe injuries to children are man-made, the side effect of the products and environments people design, build, and use. Injury prevention must become a central feature of the constructions of modern life. Along with the biggest, the sleekest, the fastest, the most convenient, and the most beautiful, the safest and the most childproof must come to be valued. Human ingenuity can come up with the solutions, but the questions need to be raised with those who do the creative thinking. Injury control needs to be taught in schools of design, architecture, and engineering.

A particular design challenge is presented by the small size of the child with respect to environments and vehicles adults and children share. Seat belts and stairways, crosswalks and appliances, indeed almost everything, has been made for the mentally and physically mature. Designs need not sacrifice the safety of the least able. Many products and architectural features which are time-honored and common present substantial injury risks for children. These need not be taken as necessary just because children have had to cope with them for generations.

Injury risk for children should be considered in the design of every new product or facility, whether or not it is intended for child use. Products intended for adults rarely can be effectively separated from children's environments, and children will enter most adult facilities at some time, such as when visiting a nursing home or workplace. Building codes for new and existing residences and other buildings should consider the needs and limitations of children. Items to be addressed include, among others, stair-handrail size and height, guardrail spacing, locking storage space, and safety glazing on accessible glass doors and windows. Model building codes do not adequately include injury-prevention strategies; the Life Safety Code of the National Fire Protection Association (NFPA) (NFPA 1988) is better than many codes for considering children's use of buildings, but there is room for improvement in that code as well. Products intended for children should be carefully scrutinized, particularly for small parts and entrapment hazards, before manufacture and marketing. If products to be marketed for children have obvious injury potential, they should never leave the drawing board. Misuse by children can be foreseen and resulting injuries eliminated by design.

There remains, in addition, a need for greater interest in creating new and improved products to protect children from foreseeable risks — helmets for sports and recreational activities, surfaces which absorb energy during a fall, car restraints for children who are prematurely born or who have deforming handicaps, and fabrics which resist ignition are only a few of the more obvious examples. Individual chapters of this book suggest many more. There are, no doubt, many designs still not dreamed of.

Underlying all these needs is the opportunity for those who design products and facilities to help sell safety — that is, to make it attractive to consumers. Safety needs to be convenient and affordable. It needs to appeal to children and their parents — no mean task and certainly a worthy challenge.

2.H Business and Industry

The best interest of the consumer is ultimately the best interest of business and industry. Safety sells from a number of perspectives. First, when the safety of child users is considered during the design phase of product development, the ultimate cost of manufacturing the product may not be increased at all. Attention to injury potential during design and testing pays off by lessening product-liability risks and by obviating the need for recall and retrofitting. Second, there remains a great opportunity for developing, manufacturing, and marketing new safety products and equipment for children. Competition in this area would be likely to stimulate new and creative solutions to pressing needs like the protection of the child's head during sporting activities. Third, contrary to popular myth, there is no reason to believe safety will not sell.

Two particular opportunities should be highlighted. Expanded strategies for premarket testing of products for their injury-producing potential would be a welcome innovation. Development of marketing approaches which successfully emphasize safety deserves attention.

Groups such as ASTM (formerly known as the American Society for Testing and Materials) and the American National Standards Institute (ANSI) develop voluntary standards which, when adhered to, provide an increased level of protection for children. Because the agendas of many different interests are balanced by these organizations, the standards promulgated do not always represent the highest level of protection which might be achieved. Advocacy for the interests of children within such organizations is always needed, as is innovation in the science of testing. Products imported from other countries may not comply with U.S. mandatory or voluntary standards. Importers must be responsible for ensuring that their products do comply with all applicable standards. The considerable expertise and data bank developed by the Consumer Product Safety Commission over the years of its existence can be of assistance to those from the business community who wish to provide leadership in the area of childhood injury prevention.

Finally, manufacturers and businesses must make certain children are not likely to be injured during the course of business. Unsupervised children should not be able to penetrate construction sites and mining operations, for instance. Priority should be given to operating the vehicles of commerce without maiming children. Places of business should be childproofed. The business practices of today greatly affect the consumers of tomorrow.

2.I Mass Media

Over the past few years, the media have increasingly featured injury as a public health problem, and this emphasis should continue. Yet the role of the media is even broader. Newspapers, magazines, radio, television, and films provide an opportunity to present, both directly and indirectly, injury-prevention messages to large numbers of people. Few, if any, segments of the population are not media consumers, so the media reach high-risk populations that do not benefit from the advocacy of some other groups. Disparate groups of professionals influence the form and content of what people read, hear, and watch. Not all will even consider themselves as wearing the "mass media" label. Few see injury prevention as their objective, yet the decisions of many affect injury risk. Three broad categories of media involvement have been used to structure the mass media sections of the specific chapters which follow: (1) key messages to be emphasized in public-service announcements or social-marketing campaigns (Manoff 1985); (2) information directed to reporters and editors; and (3) portrayal of injury-prevention measures and risks in all forms of media features and advertising.

Media messages can provide information and/or attempt to motivate behavioral change on the part of individuals or decision makers. Direct marketing of injury-prevention strategies (such as public-service announcements) may not succeed over the short term as an isolated approach. Seat belt ads, though well prepared and frequently aired, did not result in higher seat belt use, for instance (Robertson et al. 1974). Parents who viewed a television program on home hazards without other interventions did not correct the hazards (Colver et al. 1982). However, in almost every community-wide program that does succeed in increasing use of a safety strategy or decrease injury, the media have been a necessary piece of the package. Without the media hype, the health-promotion campaign to encourage seat belt use discussed in section 3.C.3 would no doubt have been weaker. Without media attention, the bicycle helmet campaigns discussed in section 6.A would have been less successful. Frequently, the ability of the media to keep an issue before the public is the key to holding the many facets of an injury-prevention campaign together through time. Media attention often builds public awareness and support for other strategies, such as legislation.

"Freak accident" is a phrase often used in reports of an event leading to injury, perhaps because emphasizing the incident as bizarre or unusual makes it more newsworthy. The cause of injury prevention would be better served by emphasizing the predictable quality of most injury-producing events and what could be done to avoid them. Consideration of preventive strategies, without "blaming the victim," could become a part of reporting an injury event. The repetition of inaccuracies and myths ("It was a good thing he was thrown from that car or he might have been hurt") by reporters can give them the aura of truth. Recognition that there are experts in the field of injury control (New England Network to Prevent Childhood Injuries 1988) should lead to calling upon their knowledge to moderate the effect of reporting lay opinion. In an investigative role, media can add to knowledge about injury causation and especially the incentives and barriers to change.

A significant impact of the media may be in the hidden message presented. If all heroes pictured in cars are wearing seat belts even when the subject has nothing to do with car safety, seat belt use may soon become the community expectation and then the standard. If children wear helmets whenever they are shown biking in print, television, or films, readers and viewers may be more likely to do so, too. If television stars settle their differences with gunfire, children may be predisposed to violence. Perhaps the most insidious way the media may contribute to injury rather than its prevention, however, is through advertising products. Accepting advertisements that encourage the use of products unsafe for children, such as all-terrain vehicles, is one example. Another blatant example is advertisements linking alcohol with the "good things" in life. Alcohol consumption is known to contribute to a significant number of events during which adults, adolescents, and children are injured. Though more difficult to measure, the influence of alcohol on parenting skills probably contributes to a large number of childhood injuries as well. All of these questions are important and worthy of research.

It is fitting to close this section as well as the chapter with a call for more study of the complex problem of childhood injury and for evaluation of those solutions currently suggested. The best decisions often come from the most complete information. Reasoned action, however, should not be delayed; too many children will suffer.

References

American Academy of Pediatrics. 1988. *Injury Prevention, Policy Statement*. Elk Grove Village, Ill.: American Academy of Pediatrics.
Baker, SP, and Waller, AE. 1989. *Childhood Injury: State-by-State Mortality Facts*. Baltimore, Md.: Johns Hopkins University Injury Prevention Center.
Baltimore Bicycling Club. 1986. Legal and Legislative Affairs Committee. *Baltimore Bicycling Newsletter* 19(2):21.
Colver, AF, et al. 1982. Promoting children's home safety. *Br Med J* 285:1177–1180.
Micik, S, et al. 1987. *Preventing Childhood Injuries: A Guide for Public Health Agencies*, (ed. 2). San Marcos, Calif.: North County Health Services.
Nader, PR. 1985. Improving the practice of pediatric patient education: A synthesis and selective review. *Prev Med* 14(6):688–701.
National Committee for Injury Prevention and Control. 1989. *Injury Prevention: Meeting the Challenge*. New York: Oxford University Press.
National Fire Protection Association. 1988. *Life Safety Code* (NFPA 101). Quincy, Mass.: National Fire Protection Association.
New England Network to Prevent Childhood Injuries. 1988. *Injury Prevention Professionals: A National Directory*. Newton, Mass.: Education Development Center.

Pless, IB, and Arsenault, L. 1987. The role of health education in the prevention of injuries to children. *Journal of Social Issues* 43(2):87–103.

Robertson, LS, et al. 1974. A controlled study of the effect of television messages on safety belt use. *Am J Public Health* 64(11):1071–1080.

Thompson, RS, et al. 1989. A case-control study of the effectiveness of bicycle safety helmets. *N Engl J Med* 320(21):1361–1367.

II

THE ROADWAY ENVIRONMENT

3

Motor Vehicle Occupants

3.A Facts

Motor vehicle-occupant injuries are a prominent cause of death for children of all ages and the leading cause of death for older children and adolescents. More than 1,600 children younger than 15 years of age are killed in motor vehicles each year in the United States, and more than 200,000 are treated in emergency departments.

The highest death rates among preteenagers occur in the very youngest children (see figure 3-1); during the first 6 months of life, the death rate is twice as high as for children aged 2-10. Beginning at about age 10, mortality increases rapidly, primarily among boys. Head injuries predominate as a cause of death, especially in the youngest children. Nonfatal injuries with serious or even devastating effects include brain and spinal cord injury and facial disfigurement.

The trauma causing most deaths and disabilities occurs a fraction of a second after a crash, when an unrestrained child strikes the vehicle interior. Proper use of car safety seats or seat belts will usually prevent injurious contact with the vehicle interior and keep the child from being ejected from the car, an often lethal event. In addition to injuries in crashes, about one-tenth of the children injured as motor vehicle occupants strike the vehicle interior during a sudden stop, turn, or swerve; such noncrash injuries may be severe and are most common among unrestrained 1- to 4-year-olds (Agran et al. 1985).

More than half of all deaths or severe injuries to motor vehicle occupants can be prevented by the use of restraints. In fact, properly used car safety seats for children appear to reduce the risk of severe injury or death in a crash by as much as 70% (Kahane 1986). Restraints of all types protect occupants by securing them to the vehicle so that their bodies stop more slowly in a crash and are less likely to be thrown against the vehicle's interior than unrestrained occupants. Restraints also are designed to spread the impact forces widely over strong parts of the body.

Car safety seats should be used until a child outgrows them and fits the vehicle's built-in restraint system well. Preference should be given to seats and seating positions providing protection against side impact as well as

Number of Deaths

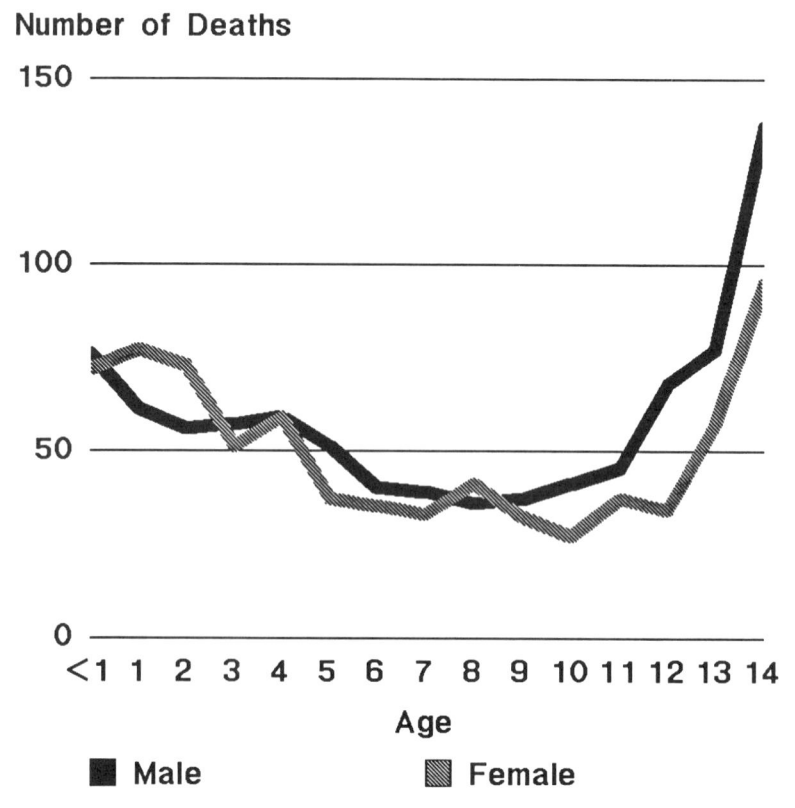

FIGURE 3-1. *Childhood motor vehicle-occupant deaths by age, U.S., 1986. (Source: National Center for Health Statistics 1988.)*

frontal crashes. Seats must be installed and used with strict attention to the manufacturer's guidelines. All car safety seats must be securely fastened to the vehicle, ideally in the rear central position, and the child must be secured within the seat. Infant safety seats must be used facing the rear window so that frontal crash forces are spread across the infant's back. Toddlers may face forward. Misuse of seats is a common and important problem, because incorrectly used seats do not provide maximum protection and may even contribute to injury. Typical errors are failure to use or incorrect routing of the vehicle's seat belt around the safety seat, failure to use the seat's harness straps or to fit them snugly to the child, placing the shoulder straps under the child's arms, or allowing the lap straps to ride up onto the abdomen because the crotch strap is too long (Weber 1989). Though there are many barriers to car seat use (Gielen et al. 1984), including cultural attitudes, it is now so widely accepted and established that failure to provide such protection may constitute neglect.

Passengers in the rear seat are better protected than passengers in the front seat in most crashes by seating position alone. A lap belt provides

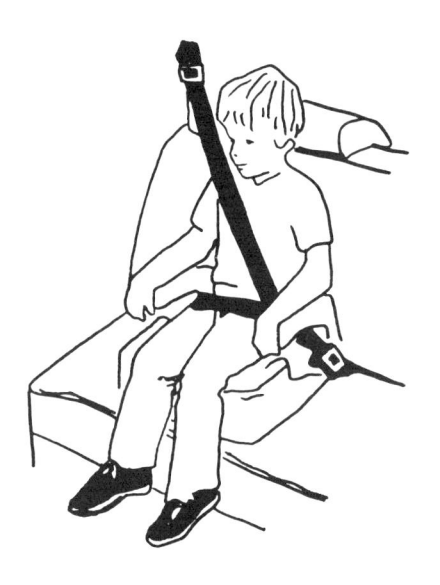

FIGURE 3-2. *Belt-positioning booster seat with three-point restraint system in place. Such seats should not be used with a lap belt alone. (From Shelness 1990. Copyright 1990 by Annemarie Shelness. Reprinted by permission.)*

additional benefits in any seating position (Kahane 1987). Even more protection is afforded by lap/shoulder (three-point) systems, which prevent the body from jackknifing and disperse the impact forces over a wider body area than do lap belts alone. These systems were not installed in the rear of most cars until recently. Three-point systems are required in cars manufactured after December 10, 1989, for all forward-facing rear "outboard" seat positions and can be retrofitted in many earlier models. Car safety seats, including infant seats which are used in the rear-facing position, can be used with a three-point system.

Seat belts can be used to restrain a small child but are not as protective as safety seats. Therefore, the laws of most states require the use of safety seats for small children. If a safety seat is not available, young children are safer using a lap belt than traveling unrestrained. Shoulder belts should be used as soon as children are tall enough that they no longer cross the face or neck.

Special arrangements must be made to restrain children who are too big for a car safety seat but too short for a shoulder belt (i.e., it crosses the face or neck). From the most acceptable to the least, the possibilities include: (1) a belt-positioning booster seat with a three-point belt system (see figure 3-2); (2) a tethered vest (which requires installing an anchor); (3) a large-shield booster; (4) a small-shield booster; or (5) a lap belt alone with the shoulder strap, if there is one, behind the child (never under the arm). At any age, a lap belt must be fastened snugly around the lap against the thighs rather than across the abdomen (see figure 3-3) to prevent belt-related injuries.

Child-restraint and seat belt laws have measurably increased restraint use, especially when vigorously enforced (Williams and Wells 1981; Campbell 1988). Laws permitting primary enforcement have been shown to be more effective than those that permit only secondary enforcement; primary

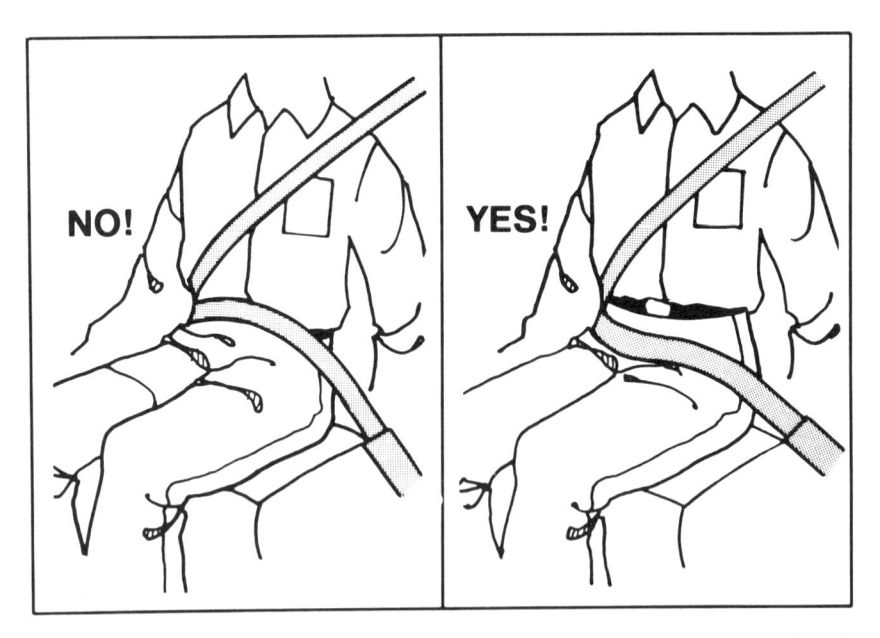

FIGURE 3-3. *Proper positioning of a three-point restraint system (lap and shoulder belts). (Courtesy of National Highway Traffic Safety Administration. Reprinted by permission.)*

enforcement allows a police officer to issue a ticket solely because of nonuse of a seat belt rather than limiting ticketing to cases involving another violation.

Air bags are inflatable cushions that provide increased protection and are strongly recommended in addition to seat belt use. They inflate automatically in potentially serious frontal crashes. They spread the impact forces over a longer period of time and a larger area of the body than belts and provide additional protection against contact with hard structures. At present, however, they are factory installed only for the driver's position in selected new cars (and in a very few models for front-seat passengers). Air bags in other positions and vehicles ordinarily require special purchase arrangements or retrofitting. Passive shoulder belts that slide into position as the car door is closed are increasingly available. When left intact, they offer the advantage of automatic protection, but users must be reminded to manually fasten the lap belt. Unfortunately, some drivers (and even some dealers) disconnect the belts so automatic protection is not provided.

Alcohol is a factor in the majority of fatal crashes and in a large proportion of serious injury crashes. No age is immune, and young teenage drivers (with whom children may be riding) are especially susceptible to the effects of alcohol. Laws raising the legal drinking age to 21 and curfew laws have reduced serious crashes involving teenage drivers (Rivara 1988; IIHS 1990a).

Other important determinants of injury to occupants include travel speed (when the crash speed doubles, the forces increase fourfold), vehicle design (e.g., subcompacts offer substantially less crash protection), and highway design (e.g., fewer fatalities occur when traffic moving in opposite directions is separated) — all factors that can be manipulated.

3.B Developmental Considerations

3.B.0 The Fetus

In the case of motor vehicle–occupant injury, risk clearly begins before birth. Car crashes are the leading cause of maternal death, which puts the fetus in obvious jeopardy. In addition, the forces sustained by the pregnant abdomen during a crash can injure the fetus or precipitate early delivery, with its additional risks. Unfortunately, though pregnancy does not contraindicate lap and shoulder belts, use falls during pregnancy, depriving both the mother and the fetus of this protection.

3.B.1 Infants

Infant motor vehicle occupants are completely dependent on the decisions of adults for protection. Traditionally, infants have been held in a parent's arms. Dynamic testing clearly shows that even a parent who is properly restrained cannot overcome the inertial forces exerted in a serious crash to maintain a grasp on a child. Therefore, the arms of an adult are not an adequate restraint device. In a crash, an unrestrained infant becomes a missile crashing into the interior of the car. The relatively large head of the infant may make it a likely contact point; head injury is common.

The infant's small size, primitive motor development, particularly the inability to sit, large head size with little muscular control at the neck, and protruding abdomen all make design of restraints a challenge. Current safety seats deal with some of these by placing the infant facing the rear of the car to allow more favorable dynamics in the common frontal collision. Infant care needs that cannot be accomplished while the infant is restrained, such as feeding and diapering, necessitate frequent stops. The ability to observe the infant while the car is in motion is also important to parents. Though installing the infant seat in the rear seat provides maximum protection, if the driver must see the child, it is preferable to use the infant seat in the rear-facing position in the front seat than to install it facing forward in the rear seat (Weber 1989).

Low-birthweight infants need special considerations when restraints are chosen because (1) their bodies may be too small for the safety seat harness system and their faces too close to a shield or lap pad, and (2) some low-birthweight infants breathe poorly in standard safety seats (see section 3.C.2).

3.B.2 Toddlers

Observation studies have shown that restraint use is lower for toddlers than for infants. The improved motor skills of toddlers (e.g., crawling, walking, and climbing) allow them to be disruptive in the car. Unrestrained toddlers are often out of position—that is, not sitting on the seat. The activities of the child may actually contribute to a crash by distracting the driver. Fortunately, observation studies show that children actually behave better in cars when properly restrained than when unrestrained (Christophersen 1977).

Developmental advances in cognition and fine motor skills and the appropriate curiosity of a toddler will allow the child at some point during this period or the next to figure out how to wriggle free of the restraint system even though the releases are designed to be difficult for a child to operate. The parent must be prepared to insist on compliance in spite of the temper tantrums so characteristic of the age.

3.B.3 Preschoolers

Current safety seats for toddlers are dynamically tested using a 35-pound dummy and are recommended for children up to a weight of about 40 pounds. The average girl reaches this weight at about 5 years, the average boy at about $4\frac{1}{2}$ years. The seat's harness system may be too tight to buckle even before the weight limit is reached (Weber 1989). Therefore, preschoolers eventually "grow out" of their car seats. Moreover, the preschooler often expresses an urgent desire to see or reach out the window and to sit in the front seat, and is quite likely to open an unlocked door, all of which may contribute to injury. It is important that children who have outgrown their car safety seats be restrained in booster seats or with carefully placed seat belts rather than be allowed to ride unrestrained (see section 3.A).

As lap belts are currently designed, they tend to ride up onto the abdomen of a preschooler who is on the seat, and most current shoulder belts are unsuitable for the truncal height of the preschooler, crossing the body at the neck or face. Out-of-position belts, while preferable to no restraints at all, can contribute to injury. A belt-positioning booster seat can be used to improve belt position.

3.B.4 Elementary School Ages

The school-age child gradually grows up to fit currently installed three-point belt systems. At this age children are quite likely to reflect family values as motor vehicle occupants, and their belt use is heavily determined by parental practices (Macknin et al. 1987).

3.B.5 Young Adolescents

During the early adolescent years, children are highly subject to pressure from peers, who may discourage seat belt use or contribute to misinformation about their value. Young adolescents may ride with older friends who have just become drivers and are in the highest crash-risk category by virtue of age. Eager to drive themselves, they may be tempted to operate a motor vehicle before licensed to do so. Alcohol use becomes a factor to be reckoned with.

3.C Opportunities for Protection

STRATEGIES FOR PREVENTING INJURIES TO MOTOR VEHICLE OCCUPANTS
(high-priority strategies are indicated by a △)

Changing the Vehicle and Equipment

△ Provide driver and passenger air bags in cars.
△ Provide three-point restraint systems that adequately protect children in the rear seating positions.
△ Design and promote cars with good crash-protection features, such as side-impact protection.
  Make retrofitting older cars with three-point restraint systems inexpensive and easy.
  Provide seats and seat belts designed to accommodate car seats properly and easily.
  Provide safety seats that are easy to use and difficult to misuse, that are comfortable for children, and that children cannot easily open.
  Develop occupant protection for passengers in the back of pickup trucks.

Increasing the Use of Safety Seats and Seat Belts

△ Pass laws requiring seat belt use by children over 4 years of age.
  Amend existing child-restraint laws to close gaps in coverage.
  Enforce safety seat and seat belt laws.
  Provide loaner and/or rental programs for safety seats.
  Encourage organizations to adopt internal regulations requiring safety seat and seat belt use for children being transported for organizational activities.

Changing the Highway Environment

△ Keep speed limits at 55 mph (or less, where appropriate).
  Provide adequate shoulders for emergency use.
  Install guardrails, "breakaway" signs, and crash-attenuating devices to reduce crash forces.
  Ensure that signs and signals provide drivers with necessary information clearly and in time to make decisions.
  Reduce likelihood of crashes with one-way streets and limited-access roads.
  Identify high-risk areas and reduce the hazards.

3.C.1 Schools and Child Care Centers

Schools should require that children who are being transported during the school hours in private vehicles (e.g., on field trips) be restrained by a seat belt and shoulder harness as appropriate for the child's size. The number of passengers should not exceed the number of restraints, and adults should also wear seat belts. Seating in the rear seat is preferable to being seated in the front seat. Day care centers that are transporting children should have a rule requiring the proper use of child safety seats and seat belts. Schools for children with special needs, including handicapping conditions, must see to their special restraint needs (see section 3.C.2).

Schools have many additional opportunities to inform children and their parents about passenger safety through standard and innovative educational techniques. Supporting materials are available (see additional sources of information). Care should be taken that all such efforts focus on the desirability of seat belts, and additionally, air bags, since tomorrow's consumers are schoolchildren today.

The installation and use of seat belts on school buses has been a matter of controversy for several years (IIHS 1985; TRB 1989). Arguments against such use have suggested that the construction of the seats and floorboards is inadequate to properly anchor seat belts, and that the backs of the seats themselves can be made higher and of energy-absorbing materials designed to obviate the need for seat belts. Others argue that training children to wear seat belts in school buses will positively influence their overall traveling behavior. Over the years, the number of children who have died as occupants in school bus crashes has been small, and resources might be directed first to assuring better protection of child pedestrians around school buses (see chapter 5).

3.C.2 Health Care Providers

Health care providers were a major force in getting child-restraint laws passed in every state. Recognizing their strength in this area, health care providers should continue their advocacy for the legislative, regulatory, and community strategies to protect motor vehicle occupants as discussed in sections 3.C.4 and 3.C.6.

Health care providers can use contacts with patients and parents as an occasion to educate them about the need to use car seat and seat belt systems consistently and correctly. Incorrect use of safety seats is very common, so health care providers must have knowledge of and advise correct usage. Studies show that health-education programs must be vigorous, make use of sound behavioral and educational principles, be repeated and sustained, and be accompanied by other strategies to bring about satisfactory usage levels (Pless and Arsenault 1987). Even then some families are unlikely to comply. This is not surprising given the fact that car seats are troublesome to use and that seats and belts must be used so many times in a car-oriented society.

Health care providers who deal with children must now focus on the car safety needs of children with special health problems, including premature infants or infants with low birthweight, children in casts, and children with various health problems, who were inadequately served in the initial efforts to get most children into restraints (see additional sources of information).

The first-choice restraint device for a low-birthweight infant is one of the available safety seats without lap pad or shield and with shoulder straps no more than 10 inches above the seat bottom and crotch strap no more than $5\frac{1}{2}$ inches from the seat back (Richards 1989). A retainer strap may be needed to keep the shoulder straps close together and around the small infant. Blankets or towels may be rolled and placed between the infant and each side of the seat. A third roll between the infant and the crotch strap is needed to prevent slouch with some models. An adult should sit beside the infant to observe respiratory status (Bull and Stroup 1985). Some premature infants develop hypoxia, bradycardia, or both in typical car seat positions (Willett et al. 1989). Before hospital discharge, babies born prematurely should be observed properly strapped and supported in the seat by a member of the medical staff. Infants who do not tolerate the position may be tried supine or prone in a seat that permits a very small angle of recline. Failing that, a specially designed restraining car bed can be obtained (Richards 1989). These are more expensive and theoretically provide less certain protection for the head in a side-impact crash, though they appear to be performing well in actual use (Weber 1989).

Special restraining arrangements and seat modifications have been developed for children with spica and body casts, for children with neuromuscular problems that prevent their sitting unassisted, and for children in wheelchairs (Richards 1989). In situations where children must be transported with heavy medical equipment, such as monitors and ventilators, the equipment must be secured as well as the child, so that it does not become a missile in the event of a crash.

Though restraint use has become a byword for primary care physicians and trauma surgeons, other health professionals might become more involved. Those seeing adults should advise belt use; this will protect not only adults but also their children, since belt use by the parent is associated with use by the child, and since death or disability of a parent has marked impact on the child. Obstetricians can approach the problem from their interest in the mother-fetus unit and dentists from their interest in preventing facial and dental problems, for example. In addition to usual health maintenance visits, health professionals may wish to present education during prenatal classes, at home visits, or as part of emergency visits for injury.

Health professionals working as a group have been able to bring about greatly increased car seat use at hospital discharge by providing hospital-based rental programs (Colletti 1986). Hospitals should develop and adhere to policies requiring that all newborns and pediatric patients leaving the hospital in a car or truck be protected in a car safety seat (Decker et al. 1988). Hospitals and health care providers also have a special obligation to assure adequate restraint of children riding in emergency vehicles and to advocate access to emergency care in currently underserved rural areas.

The health care community has yet to address, by any intervention, the fact that for many children injured in a crash related to alcohol the drinking driver was their own parent.

3.C.3 Public Agencies

All agencies that transport children should have internal rules requiring the use of seat belts, car seats, or special restraints, as appropriate to the age and condition of the child. Agencies that have opportunities to interact with parents of young children should promote the use of seat belts and car seats, including the provision of loaner and/or sale programs for car seats.

Using car seats to protect children from injury is becoming part of the minimum standard for child care in America. A significant proportion of the parent population, however, regularly fails to meet this standard (and an even larger proportion fails to do so occasionally). This failure may be appropriately considered evidence of neglect. Like all other forms of neglect, failure to use car safety seats should be approached with a mixture of education (e.g., media campaigns), practical support (e.g., getting hospitals, preschools, and day care centers to loan them as necessary), and enforcement (e.g., instructing police to be active and aggressive in issuing summonses to violators, with penalties contingent upon compliance, and special efforts directed at repeat offenders).

One health-promotion campaign aimed at promoting seat belt use throughout the community enlisted the cooperation of multiple community resources and successfully increased observed use of seat belts (Gemmings et al. 1984). Interested agencies might consider similar cooperative campaigns.

3.C.4 Legislators and Regulators

All 50 states and the District of Columbia have laws requiring very young children to be restrained in cars. However, the laws vary widely from state to state on such factors as the age of the children covered by the law, the type of vehicle, and the relationship between the driver and the child. Most of the state laws cover only very young children; many states no longer require the use of any restraint by the age children begin school (Teret et al. 1986). State laws should require that children who have outgrown child-restraint devices be restrained by seat belts. Even in states with seat belt laws, older children may be unprotected since the laws may be limited to front-seat outboard positions.

Other gaps in coverage need to be closed through amendments to existing laws. For example, some states exempt pickup trucks from coverage even though a large percentage of the child occupants killed in those states were riding in pickup trucks. Many state laws require compliance only from child occupants riding with their parents, and many laws apply only to vehicles registered in the state.

A uniform law has been developed to provide the greatest possible coverage to child occupants of motor vehicles (see additional sources of information). State legislators should compare their state's law with that contained in the Uniform Vehicle Code; where the state's law is less stringent, it should be amended to conform to the uniform law. For maximum effectiveness, all restraint laws should allow for primary enforcement.

Many fatal crashes involving young drivers occur at night (Robertson and Zador 1978). In order to reduce the likelihood that children and adolescents will be injured as occupants in cars being driven unsafely by older siblings or friends, legislatures can pass curfew laws (IIHS 1984, 1990a) and can issue limited-hour licenses to young drivers (Preusser et al. 1984). Laws limiting speeds to 55 mph have been shown to reduce the likelihood of serious injuries (Baker et al. 1984). Similarly, optimum vehicle design and improved road characteristics, often influenced by regulation, will reduce injuries to occupants of all ages. New vehicle designs, like the multipurpose vehicles now popular for family transportation, should swiftly be made to conform to Department of Transportation standards for passenger safety promulgated for passenger cars.

Traffic slows when detectable radar signals are present (Pezoldt and Brackett 1988), suggesting that radar detectors influence speed. The manufacture, sale, purchase, and use of these devices, which are intended only to allow drivers to break the law without being apprehended, should be illegal.

3.C.5 Law Enforcement Professionals

Enforcement of child-restraint laws and seat belt laws is the key to their success. Rank-and-file police personnel, who have the opportunity to enforce these laws, should be educated to recognize their importance. Commendations for active enforcement practices can serve as an incentive. Safety seat and seat belt misuse is a major concern; misuse detection training can be mandated.

Some occupant-protection laws provide only for secondary enforcement, meaning that drivers can be ticketed for a violation only if they have first been stopped for violating another law. In states with such secondary-enforcement laws, police should give advice to persons with unrestrained children as permitted within the intent of the law, even if they cannot be cited. Police managers should develop incentives for officers to do so.

Law enforcement personnel should be required to wear their own seat belts when they drive or ride. Their importance as role models and authorities on road safety is often overlooked. Seat belts and car seats should be available and used by passengers in police vehicles. Police have also testified in favor of occupant-protection laws, primary enforcement, 55-mph speed limits, and laws banning radar detectors.

3.C.6 Voluntary Organizations

Provision of convenient, affordable car safety seat rental programs is an important contribution of voluntary organizations to child passenger safety. Technical assistance manuals are available (see additional sources of information). Many rental programs concentrate their efforts on infant restraints; seats appropriate for the toddler should also be provided.

In communities where car seat programs have already been established, publicity campaigns must be planned for intervals to support sustained use; how frequently reminders are needed has yet to be established, however. Health-promotion campaigns organized on a community level that provide incentives (like prizes) and broadly based educational messages can increase seat belt use (Gemming et al. 1984). Reinforcement campaigns should follow at intervals to sustain gains in usage. The fact that car seat use for infants exceeds seat belt use in older children suggests groups interested in child passenger safety should address this transition directly.

Organizations and clubs that transport children in private vehicles should make and enforce regulations requiring restraint use.

Community groups can play an important role in identifying hazardous roads and especially dangerous spots where crashes have occurred or are likely to occur. Rectifying such problems is possible once they are identified and publicized.

3.C.7 Designers, Architects, Builders, and Engineers

Though design changes have made car seats easier to use, further efforts can be made to (1) simplify use and minimize misuse, (2) reduce cost, and (3) improve protection. At least one adult passenger seat has been developed with a built-in, fold-down restraint system that transforms to accommodate infants and larger children (IIHS 1989). Such built-in devices could solve many access and misuse problems and could facilitate crash testing.

Very small infants, especially those prematurely born, may not breathe properly in a safety seat unless special care is taken to prop them in such a way that their heads do not droop, blocking the airway; special design modifications are needed and are beginning to appear. At least one car bed restraint is now available to restrain infants lying down; further innovations in this area are welcome. Also important, restraint systems have yet to be designed for many groups of children with handicaps (Richards 1989) (see section 3.C.2).

Seat belt systems should be designed to accommodate the use of a car seat without special modification. More attention needs to be directed toward design changes that would make belt systems safer and more effective for the preschool and school-age child. Automatic belt systems should be tested for protection of the child. Air bags and other forms of automatic protection, such as side-impact protection, should be provided for all seating positions. Passenger-car safety standards should be applied to the design of minivans and light trucks.

Modifications of vehicle design that decrease the likelihood that the passenger compartment will be violated in a crash will decrease injury to children, both restrained and unrestrained, and further modifications of design and materials, like nonlacerating windshields, will reduce injury.

Roadway modifications that decrease speed (e.g., speed bumps, culs-de-sac in residential areas) decrease the likelihood of crashes. Separation of traffic lanes on thoroughfares (e.g., wide medians, one-way traffic) and limited-access roads decrease crashes and therefore injuries.

3.C.8 Business and Industry

Manufacturers now recognize that consumers will pay for safety (IIHS 1990b). Crashworthiness and restraint systems are a marketing plus. Manufacturers can encourage dealers to make safety seats or safety-seat information available to consumers, to show cars with automatic belts connected, and to require appropriate restraints during a test drive. Reaching consumers with recall notices for modification of safety-seat problems has been cumbersome and inadequate. Improvements, possibly including a registration system, are needed.

Though admittedly not yet a strategy for protecting passengers in the rear seat, where many children sit, the adoption of air bags for front seat occupants is a step toward providing protection for all. The benefits and proven safety record of air bags have not become common knowledge. Myths about lack of efficacy and inadvertent deployment need to be countered with facts. Automobile manufacturers should make dealers familiar with air-bag technology, safety, and efficacy, should help dealers become knowledgeable about which models include air bags as standard equipment, and should encourage dealers to promote them. Manufacturers and dealers can turn air bags, as well as other safety features, into a positive marketing strategy.

The insurance industry can expand programs to increase insurance benefits or decrease costs to consumers who own vehicles with automatic restraints or who use restraints and to penalize drivers with radar detectors (IIHS 1988). Other businesses can encourage the use of seat belts and safety seats by their employees and their families through informational campaigns and programs to reward use. At least one company gives employees who are new parents a safety seat as a gift. Parental seat belt use is a strong predictor of children's seat belt use. Employers are likely to benefit by experiencing fewer lost workdays and lower benefit costs. In addition, businesses can donate safety seats to rental programs.

The role of toy manufacturers in increasing the acceptability of safety seats and seat belts might be explored. Restraint systems could be provided in toys and pictured in use in industry-sponsored programming for children. If dolls and superhero figures ride restrained, perhaps children will expect to do so, too.

3.C.9 Mass Media

Evaluations show that a media campaign, *combined with* enforcement of seat belt laws, results in an increase in seat belt use (IIHS 1987). The most effective pattern may be an initial blitz followed by short reinforcing campaigns at intervals (Williams et al. 1987), but further evaluation of this marketing strategy would be helpful.

Members of the news media need to be accurately informed about the causes of motor vehicle-occupant injury so that misinformation and uninformed opinion—for example, a prevalent myth: "It's lucky he was thrown from the car"—are not inadvertently supported by repetition in news stories. Also, editors should direct attention appropriate to the size of the problem to the issue of motor vehicle-occupant injury. For example, 33,629 Americans died in battle in the Korean War and 47,356 in the Vietnam War. By comparison, 47,093 Americans died in motor vehicle crashes during 1988 alone. Media attention could be used to help change the fatalistic attitude many people have about motor vehicle injuries and to stress the idea that these injuries can and should be prevented (Rivara 1988).

Whenever possible, people in programs and ads should be pictured riding appropriately restrained; celebrities can make a particular impact on children. Advertisements that promote speed should be avoided. The misinformation conveyed by programs showing high-speed chases needs to be reduced *and* combated with realistic information on the injuries likely to result from such activities.

References

Agran, PF, et al. 1985. Noncrash motor vehicle accidents: Injuries to children in the vehicle interior. *Am J Dis Child* 139(3):304-306.

Baker, SP, et al. 1984. *The Injury Fact Book*. Lexington, Mass.: Lexington Books.

Bull, MJ, and Stroup, KB. 1985. Premature infants in car seats. *Pediatrics* 75(2): 336-339.

Campbell, BJ. 1988. The association between enforcement and seat belt use. *Journal of Safety Research* 19(4):159-163.

Campbell, BJ, et al. 1984. *The Use of Economic Incentives and Public Education to Increase Seat Belt Use in a Community*. Chapel Hill, N.C.: University of North Carolina Highway Safety Research Center.

Christophersen, ER. 1977. Children's behavior during automobile rides: Do car seats make a difference? *Pediatrics* 60(1):69-74.

Colletti, RB. 1986. Longitudinal evaluation of a statewide network of hospital programs to improve child passenger safety. *Pediatrics* 77(4):523-529.

Decker, MD, et al. 1988. Failure of hospitals to promote the use of child restraint devices. *Am J Dis Child* 142(6):656.

Gemming, MG, et al. 1984. A community health education approach to occupant protection. *Health Educ Q* 11(2):147-158.

Gielen, AC, et al. 1984. Factors associated with the use of child restraint devices. *Health Educ* 11(2):195-206.

Insurance Institute for Highway Safety. 1979. *Status Report* 14(18).

Insurance Institute for Highway Safety. 1984. *Status Report* 19(10).

Insurance Institute for Highway Safety. 1985. Special issue: School buses and seat belts. *Status Report* 20(5).

Insurance Institute for Highway Safety. 1987. What kind of campaign promotes the highest belt law compliance? *Status Report* 22(13):5.
Insurance Institute for Highway Safety. 1988. GEICO appeal. *Status Report* 23(7): 2.
Insurance Institute for Highway Safety. 1989. New child restraint protects child from birth to age of 10. *Status Report* 24(8):6.
Insurance Institute for Highway Safety. 1990a. Curfew laws reduce traffic injuries to teenagers 23 percent. *Status Report* 25(1):3.
Insurance Institute for Highway Safety. 1990b. Allstate award. *Status Report* 25(1):4.
Kahane, CJ. 1986. *An Evaluation of Child Passenger Safety: The Effectiveness and Benefits of Safety Seats.* NHTSA Report No. DOT HS 806 890. Washington, D.C.: U.S. Dept. of Transportation.
Kahane, CJ. 1987. *Fatality and Injury Reducing Effectiveness of Lap Belts for Back Seat Occupants.* NHTSA Evaluation Notes. Washington, D.C.: U.S. Dept. of Transportation.
Macknin, ML, et al. 1987. Office education by pediatricians to increase seat belt use. *Am J Dis Child* 141:1305–1307.
National Center for Health Statistics. 1988. *Vital Statistics of the United States, 1986.* Vol. 2, Mortality, pt. A. Dept. of Health and Human Services publication No. (PHS) 88-1122. Washington, D.C.: U.S. Government Printing Office.
Pezoldt, VJ, and Brackett, RQ. 1988. *The Impact of Radar Detectors on Highway Traffic Safety.* Washington, D.C.: National Highway Traffic Safety Administration.
Pless, IB, and Arsenault, L. 1987. The role of health education in the prevention of injuries to children. *Journal of Social Issues* 43(2):87–103.
Preusser, DF, et al. 1984. The effect of curfew laws on motor vehicle crashes. *Law and Policy* 6:115–128.
Richards, DD. 1989. The challenge of transporting children with special needs. *Safe Ride News* 8(2):1 (special insert).
Rivara, FP. 1988. Motor vehicle injuries during adolescence. *Pediatr Ann* 17(2): 107–113.
Robertson, LS, and Zador, PI. 1978. Driver education and fatal crash involvement of teenaged drivers. *Am J Public Health* 68:959.
Shelness, AM. 1990. *Don't Risk Your Child's Life.* New Milford, Conn.: Shelness Productions.
Teret, SP, et al. 1986. Child restraint laws: An analysis of gaps in coverage. *Am J Public Health* 76(1):31–34.
Transportation Research Board. 1989. *Improving School Bus Safety.* Washington, D.C.: Transportation Research Board.
Weber, K. 1989. *Automobile Restraint Systems for Children: Theory and Practice.* Paper presented at the Third National Conference on Pediatric Trauma, Ann Arbor, Mich., September 1989.
Willett, LD, et al. 1989. Ventilatory changes in convalescent infants positioned in car seats. *J Pediatr* 115:451–455.
Williams, AF, and Wells, JK. 1981. The Tennessee child restraint law in its third year. *Am J Public Health* 71(2):163–165.
Williams, AF, et al. 1987. Seat belt use law enforcement and publicity in Elmira, New York: A reminder campaign. *Am J Public Health* 77(11):1450–1451.

Additional Sources of Information

American Academy of Pediatrics (AAP)
141 Northwest Point Boulevard
PO Box 927
Elk Grove Village, IL 60009
312-228-5005
 Information on occupant protection, including *Family Shopping Guide* (for safety seats and booster seats), First Ride, Safe Ride Campaign, *Car Seat Advocacy Kit*.

American Automobile Association (AAA)
Foundation for Traffic Safety
1730 M Street, NW
Suite 401
Washington, DC 20036
202-775-1456
 Educational materials and reports.

Association for the Advancement of Automotive Medicine (AAAM)
2340 Des Plaines River Road
Suite 106
Des Plaines, IL 60018
708-390-8927
 Reports on road-related injuries.

Automotive Safety for Children Program
Riley Hospital for Children
702 Barnhill Drive, S-139
Indianapolis, IN 46223
317-274-2977
 Reference manual on special needs transportation, videotapes, other materials on occupant protection.

Highway Safety Research Center
University of North Carolina
CB #3430
Chapel Hill, NC 27599
919-962-2202
 Educational materials and reports, including *A Guide for Establishing a Car Safety Seat Rental Program*.

Insurance Institute for Highway Safety (IIHS)
1005 North Glebe Road
Suite 800
Arlington, VA 22201
703-247-1500
 Various reports on occupant protection, vehicle and roadway design.

International Association of Chiefs of Police
1110 North Glebe Road
Suite 200
Arlington, VA 22201
 Information on highway safety for law enforcement professionals.

National Committee on Uniform Traffic Laws and Ordinances
Book Department
405 Church Street
PO Box 1409
Evanston, IL 60204
800-323-4011
 Uniform Vehicle Code and Model Traffic Ordinances, 1987 edition.

National Highway Traffic Safety Administration (NHTSA)
400 7th Street, SW
Washington, DC 20590
NHTSA Toll-Free Auto Safety Hotline:
800-424-9393
 Various materials on traffic safety and safety-seat promotion, including *Early Rider Loan-A-Seat Program Manual*, *National Child Passenger Safety Awareness Week Manual* (includes list of educational materials), and updates of car-seat recall notices.

National Transportation Safety Board (NTSB)
800 Independence Avenue, SW
Washington, DC 20594
202-382-6600
 Various safety studies and crash investigations.

Note: The National Child Passenger Safety Association (NCPSA) and Physicians for Automotive Safety (PAS) are now defunct.

Society of Automotive Engineers (SAE)
400 Commonwealth Drive
Warrendale, PA 15096
412-776-4970

Technical reports on occupant protection and other aspects of motor vehicle safety, including anthropometric data for product design.

4

Users of Other Motor Vehicles

4.A Facts

Motorcycles, mopeds, minibikes, minicycles, trail bikes, snowmobiles, all-terrain vehicles (ATVs), and farm machinery share important characteristics. These vehicles provide little or no user protection. Many are unstable and apt to overturn. Often they are heavy and have the potential to reach high speeds, so the forces involved in any mishap may be substantial and the injuries correspondingly severe. Children often operate these vehicles before they are licensed to drive a car. Except for farm machinery deaths, older children (aged 10–14 years) are most often involved.

Motorcycles are usually thought of as vehicles for adults. No states license motorcycle drivers younger than 14 years old, and most do not license them younger than 16. Nevertheless, about 100 children die each year in motorcycle crashes; half are listed as the drivers. Nonfatal injuries number about 6,500 annually in the under-15 age-group, with the highest rates at ages 10–14. Leg injuries are the most common severe injuries and often are permanently disabling. Head injuries cause the largest number of deaths.

People who borrow motorcycles from friends have a high rate of crashes (Barry 1970), suggesting inexperience is a factor, and the tendency to borrow may be great among youngsters. While there are no motorcycles that should be considered safe for children to operate, high-powered racing-design motorcycles are especially hazardous, having rates of death and severe injury that are twice the rates of other motorcycles. Being carried as a rider also exposes children to a risk of death or severe injury that is far greater than the risk when traveling in a car.

Protective and reflective clothing and helmets are a must for motorcyclists of any age. Helmet laws have reduced motorcyclist deaths by 30% (Watson et al. 1980); the likelihood of nonfatal head injury also decreases with helmet use. Most states that have repealed helmet laws for adults continue to require helmets for motorcyclists younger than 18; however, in such states, many minors ride without them. Some protection to the legs of motorcycle drivers could be provided by a fenderlike structure in front of the knees, but passengers' legs are exposed to fractures and severe abrasions from sideswipes or skidding, especially on gravel.

Mopeds, minibikes, minicycles, and trail bikes typically have less-powerful engines than motorcycles but are capable of speeds of 30 mph or more. Such vehicles can be confused easily, and data for them are often grouped. Each year, more than 13,000 children are treated in emergency rooms because of injuries associated with these vehicles.

In most states, mopeds (bicycles with motors) can be ridden in traffic legally; licensure laws vary, but among those that specify mopeds the minimum age ranges from 13 to 17 years old (U.S. DOT 1988). Collisions with motor vehicles carry a high chance of death or severe injury for the moped rider. Visibility is often a factor, suggesting the need for improvements in bike lighting systems in addition to helmets and protective clothing.

Minibikes, trail bikes, and similar small cycles designed for off-road use are not regulated by federal motor vehicle safety standards, and most states require neither the rider nor the vehicle to be licensed. The rate of injuries per 100 vehicles is four times as high for minibikes as for bicycles (Rivara 1982).

Snowmobiles are a common source of injury in the winter, associated with about 2,000 injuries to children annually. Most states where snowmobiling is common require snowmobiles to be registered with some department (motor vehicles, natural resources, or other). Driver licensing is less thorough; most states allow children under a given age to operate snowmobiles on public lands as long as they are accompanied by an adult or have passed a safety training course. Head injuries are the major cause of death, with drowning also a hazard in areas where snowmobiles are used on frozen lakes. Poor stability can lead to loss of control on bumps. Snowmobiles share with ATVs and other off-road vehicles the possibility of the rider striking low branches or cables across the path, with the potential for severe or fatal injury of the neck, face, or head. Facial fractures are common, often occurring when the snowmobile is suddenly stopped by an obstacle. Though less often life threatening than injuries to the head, the largest number of injuries are to the legs. Recommendations include helmets, face and leg protection, and restricting or closely supervising use by children.

All-terrain vehicles are three- or four-wheeled vehicles designed mainly for recreational or agricultural off-road use. Licensing is not required in most states. In 1986, almost 30,000 children aged 5 to 14 were injured while riding ATVs. Head and spinal cord injuries are often disabling or even fatal. Injuries to the extremities are severe as well as common.

Designed to travel at speeds of 30 mph or greater, many ATVs have no rear-wheel differential and therefore are hard to turn, requiring unusual "body English" to do so. They overturn easily, especially on rough terrain. Concern about instability and resulting injuries led to a ban on the sale of three-wheeled ATVs in the United States in December 1987 (CPSC 1987). However, many remain in use. Injury rates are also high for four-wheeled ATVs, which can flip end over end. Four-wheelers are very heavy and therefore especially injurious when they land on top of a child rider. The fact that they were not banned should not be considered evidence that they are safe. In fact, manufacturers also agreed to take efforts to prevent the sale of adult-size, four-wheeled ATVs for use by children. Uniform compliance by dealers, however, cannot be assured; one study (Ford 1989) found that more than half of the dealers questioned continued to recommend large ATVs for children, despite the manufacturers' agreement.

Even without turning over, ATVs can cause severe injury; for example, a child may stop with an outstretched foot, allowing the rear wheel to run up the back of the leg and the rider to flip. Riding double is especially hazardous. Although ATVs are marketed for off-road use, many severe injuries and deaths occur on the highway, where their use is particularly problematic because of handling characteristics of the roadway, poor visibility, lack of protection for the riders, and the presence of other, heavier vehicles.

Data support a strong recommendation that ATV use by children younger than 16 years be prohibited (Pick 1987), and model state laws include this provision (AAP 1989). Certainly, adult-size ATVs (engine sizes greater than 90 cc) should not be used by children younger than 16, as ATV manufacturers themselves have agreed (CPSC 1987). Helmets offer protection against head injury and should be required, but cannot prevent spinal cord injury.

Farm machines are a major source of childhood death and disabling injury in agricultural states; the highest rates are in Idaho, South Dakota, Wisconsin, Vermont, Iowa, and Minnesota (Baker and Waller 1989). About 70 children are killed by farm machinery every year, and more than 4,000 are injured severely enough to require emergency room or hospital treatment. The machines most often involved in childhood injury are tractors, farm wagons, corn pickers, forklifts, tillage equipment, and conveyors (Swanson et al. 1987; Rivara 1985).

Almost three-fourths of all deaths are related to tractors (Rivara 1985). About half of all deaths occur in the 1- to 4-year age-group. Most commonly, a child is riding a tractor with a parent or other caretaker, falls off, and is crushed by the tractor or the equipment it is pulling (McKnight 1984).

Augers, while less frequently a cause of death than some farm machines, also pose a major hazard to young children, who may not understand the danger when they are playing in or near grain being moved by auger. In some farm areas, augers are the leading cause of traumatic amputation in children.

Older children are killed or injured as operators in tractor rollovers or falls from tractors, or when their clothing or body parts become entangled in unguarded power take-offs.

Thus far, farm safety programs have not solved these problems. Most interventions are particularly difficult because of the economic pressures farm families face (Wilkerson 1988). Roll-over-protective structures (ROPS) are now provided on virtually all new tractors, but retrofitting to older tractors is also an issue. Designs that would protect children are needed for parents who must carry young children when they are operating tractors (for example, a ROPS plus an enclosed compartment with a child-restraint system). Machinery redesign is needed to reduce exposure to hazardous moving parts and to prevent removal of guards.

4.B Developmental Considerations

4.B.1, 4.B.2, and 4.B.3 Infants, Toddlers, and Preschoolers

Infants and young children do not have the motor skills to operate a motor vehicle; therefore, they are injured as passengers or bystanders. Most of these vehicles are not designed to carry passengers, and none is designed to protect them. Motor vehicles are particularly inappropriate for the very young.

4.B.4 Elementary School Ages

Some motor vehicles have been sized and marketed for even the very young school-age child. Children of this age love speed and love to imitate adults, and so find motor vehicles quite attractive "toys." School-age children most often do not have the perceptual-motor skills, judgment, and experience to manage a traffic environment or rough terrain and rarely possess the skill to meet the challenge of handling an unstable vehicle consistently (Pick 1987). They are not abstract thinkers and fail to predict consequences accurately.

4.B.5 Young Adolescents

Preadolescent males are highly visible in the injury statistics from motor vehicles designed for off-road use. Eagerness to assume adult roles is typical of the age-group and may even be seen by parents as desirable—for example, in rural families where young adolescents are needed to work on the farm. At 10-12 years of age, 65% of farm boys and 23% of girls operate a tractor (Tevis and Finck 1989). While operating cars and trucks is prohibited by law, the opportunity to operate another motor vehicle probably may be seen by many children, especially boys of this age, as role enhancing and very difficult to forego. Peer pressure is strong. Statistics for passenger-car crashes suggest that 16-year-olds are less able than older persons to operate a car safely in a traffic environment. Though this is indirect evidence, it suggests that many or most preadolescents lack the skills to operate unstable but speedy vehicles on difficult terrain, also a demanding task.

4.C Opportunities for Protection

> STRATEGIES FOR PREVENTING INJURIES TO USERS OF OTHER MOTOR VEHICLES
> (high-priority strategies are indicated by a △)
>
> *Changing the Vehicle and Equipment*
> △ Provide better leg protection during crashes.
> △ Provide helmets that offer the greatest amount of protection possible.
> △ Improve safety features of new farm machinery and retrofit old with ROPS and shields for moving parts.
> Eliminate passenger seating positions on off-road vehicles.
>
> *Changing the Social Environment*
> △ Require the use of helmets.
> Place age restrictions on the use of ATVs, mopeds, snowmobiles, and farm machinery.
> Provide adequate care facilities for young children of farming families at times when the adults are operating equipment.

4.C.1 Schools and Child Care Centers

Schools can regulate the use of motor vehicles on school grounds. Prohibition of the use of mopeds, ATVs, snowmobiles, and other motor vehicles should be considered, particularly for schools in areas with dense traffic. In high-use areas, schools can educate children and parents about the injuries associated with these vehicles and can encourage riders to wear helmets.

Schools and child care providers can offer an important service in agricultural communities. Small children often are injured in falls from tractors while the tractor is being operated by a parent. The provision of adequate child care during plowing, planting, and harvesting seasons can provide young children with a safer environment than the lap of the parent driving the tractor. Educational materials on farm safety are available for schools that include agriculture in the curriculum (see additional sources of information). Farm safety should be standard in rural schools.

4.C.2 Health Care Providers

Groups of health care providers have played an important role in limiting future injuries from ATVs by urging the Consumer Product Safety Commission to act. In a court-approved agreement with the government announced in December 1987, manufacturers agreed to stop producing and selling three-wheeled ATVs in the United States. Strong resolutions and testimony from a number of physicians' groups helped move this process to fruition.

Since children younger than 16 are also at risk when operating other off-road motor vehicles (dirt bikes, four-wheeled ATVs, snowmobiles, etc.), health care provider organizations can press for voluntary agreements or legislation to prevent their sale to or use by young children. A poorer alternative is to press for legislation requiring helmet use, licensure, and training.

Health care providers should actively counsel parents *not* to provide motor vehicles for their preadolescent children. Parents who choose to allow their children to drive motor vehicles should provide instruction from an experienced adult rider; should supervise use; should insist on the use of a helmet and clothing that protects the extremities; and should prohibit carrying a passenger, night riding, and riding on the roadway or on rough terrain. When treating a child with an injury associated with a motor vehicle, its use should not be condoned. Counseling is in order to prevent future injury.

Parents who operate off-road vehicles should be discouraged from carrying child passengers. Drivers and passengers should wear helmets. In farming communities, information about childhood injuries associated with farm machinery as well as other farming-related injuries (see chapters 8, 9, 11, and 17) might be given to families by health care providers. Fact sheets and other materials are available (see additional sources of information).

4.C.3 Public Agencies

Too little is known about the occurrence and causes of injuries from non-automobile motor vehicles and about the use of these vehicles by children. Agencies can collect and analyze data on injuries and use so that preventive strategies can be formulated.

Though operation of motor vehicles by children should not be encouraged, off-road operation on designated, specially prepared trails while wearing a helmet is preferred over operation under less controlled circumstances. Agencies can provide resources to convert riders from uncontrolled to controlled riding situations, but should avoid attracting new riders.

Agencies and voluntary organizations working with farm families can make childhood injury prevention a high-priority issue. In addition to educational efforts, incentives to help farmers modify hazardous equipment and practices should be considered. Public agencies can help farmers find and afford child care for their young children during the heavy labor seasons and can help rural communities establish rescue units and train first responders (Tevis 1990).

4.C.4 Legislators and Regulators

The design of motor vehicles such as motorcycles, mopeds, snowmobiles, and ATVs can be modified through performance standards set by regulatory agencies. Leg protection from side impact is one area that deserves attention.

Legislatures can require helmet use by the young operators and passengers of these vehicles. Requiring buyers to purchase a helmet along with the vehicle might improve compliance. Helmet construction can be regulated so that the helmet provides the greatest amount of protection biomechanically possible at a reasonable cost.

Licensing requirements for operators should be considered by legislatures. Items to be considered before permitting young children to operate these motor vehicles include the dynamics of the vehicle itself, the match of the vehicle's demands to the motor skills of children of particular ages, and where the vehicle is to be operated (for example, on public thoroughfares or off-road and on steep versus level terrain). Time restrictions, such as daytime-only licenses, can also be considered.

Due to their power and instability, some vehicles are too hazardous to be operated by young persons under any circumstances (Pick 1987). All-terrain vehicles constitute a serious hazard for young persons, and the operation of either three- or four-wheeled ATVs might be legislatively banned until the age at which adolescents are licensed to drive cars.

4.C.5 Law Enforcement Professionals

Enforcement of helmet laws and age, place (e.g., off-road), and time (e.g., provisional daytime-only driver's licenses) restrictions on the operation of certain vehicles is essential. Law enforcement officers, particularly those in suburban and rural areas, where the use of motor vehicles by children is more common than in urban areas, should be educated about injury risks to young operators of motor vehicles and the need for enthusiastic enforcement of measures designed to prevent these injuries. Traffic laws apply to all vehicles used on public roads and should be enforced. Law enforcement professionals might also testify in favor of helmet laws and other measures known to reduce rider injury.

4.C.6 Voluntary Organizations

While voluntary organizations might provide training and appropriate off-road sites for children operating motor vehicles and thereby hope to decrease injuries, any gains might be offset if the services attract more riders and thus increase the number of children exposed to injury. Groups might work to make recreational use of nonmotor vehicles, such as bicycles, a more attractive and safe alternative (see also section 4.C.3). Voluntary organizations in rural areas can be instrumental in starting a community rescue unit, training volunteers, and preparing a community map so emergency medical personnel can find the correct home when needed (Tevis 1990).

4.C.7 Designers, Architects, Builders, and Engineers

Off-road vehicle designs should limit speed and maximize stability. A design standard could be introduced limiting ATVs to a top speed of 25 mph, and more stringent standards for lateral and longitudinal stability could be developed (Jagger 1990). Size and other design features should discourage use by and marketing to young children. Off-road vehicles should not be designed with a passenger seat. Leg protection could be improved by vehicle design in many cases. The muffler systems of some motorized bicycles are exposed in such a way that operators are frequently burned; design changes are needed. Designs for riding gear to protect the head, face, and legs should be continuously updated to provide the maximum protection possible given current knowledge and technology.

Moving parts of farm machinery should be shielded in such a way that body parts and clothing cannot become trapped. Modifications will be acceptable only if they do not significantly slow the process of farming. Protective guards should not be easily removed. Attention should be given to designing guards and protective devices that can be retrofitted to existing machinery where hazards have been identified. Warning labels for farm machinery should be designed to show graphically the hazards involved.

4.C.8 Business and Industry

Voluntary standards for off-road vehicles could prohibit direct or indirect marketing and sales to children, thereby decreasing the need for more formal measures. Recall of designs shown to be particularly apt to cause childhood injury (e.g., three-wheeled ATVs), in addition to suspension of sales, would help to prevent additional injuries. The ATV manufacturers' agreement to prevent the sale of adult-size four-wheeled ATVs to children and to display safety information could be strengthened by including dealers in the agreement and ensuring dealer compliance (Ford 1989). Labeling and marketing materials could clearly state that off-road vehicles are *not* appropriate for children, and new models should not be developed and marketed for children.

Education and training programs sponsored by manufacturers for child riders may be a tempting strategy. However, it is highly unlikely that children can be trained to ride these vehicles in a way that precludes injury. Educational programs must be monitored to determine if they have the insidious effect of attracting children to the vehicles, thereby increasing sales, ridership, and consequently the number of injuries.

New protective devices for existing farm machinery and new designs that provide additional safety during operation should be promoted by manufacturers and dealers. Pictorial warning labels that clearly emphasize hazards to children should be used consistently on farm machinery.

Employers in rural communities can adopt policies of flexible schedules and liberal leave time during peak farming periods so parents employed off the farm are able to supervise their children. Employer-sponsored day care is another way to keep children away from the hazards of farm machinery during periods of intense use.

4.C.9 Mass Media

Even acknowledging occasional media attention to ATVs, the injury risks for children who ride motor vehicles have been grossly underpublicized. The message needs to be that operating a motor vehicle is dangerous—far too dangerous for a child. A secondary message may be that if the first message is ignored, and a child is allowed to operate or ride such a vehicle, the child should wear a helmet and the riding should take place under extremely restrictive conditions.

Message construction will need to be particularly skillful to counteract the appeal of these "first vehicles" for children who, like their parents, are in love with power and speed. Since motor vehicles are "big-ticket" items, public health campaigns and targeted public-service announcements might concentrate air and print time before the December holidays, when these vehicles will probably be heavily advertised.

More than most sources of childhood injuries, motor vehicles are subject to seasonality, geographical variation, and waves of popularity. For these reasons, messages must be tailored to a wide variety of media markets, many of which will be rural and small. Because of the variety of vehicle types and variations in usage patterns, consultation with public health personnel will be particularly useful.

Producers and photographers should avoid showing children operating motor vehicles. When such shots are indispensable, all riders should be pictured wearing helmets.

References

American Academy of Pediatrics. 1989. *Model Bill*. Elk Grove Village, Ill.: American Academy of Pediatrics.

Baker, SP, and Waller, AE. 1989. *Childhood Injury: State-by-State Mortality Facts*. Baltimore, Md.: Johns Hopkins University Injury Prevention Center.

Barry, PZ. 1970. The role of inexperience in motorcycle crashes. *Journal of Safety Research* 2(4):229–239.

Consumer Product Safety Commission. 1987. *Statement of Terrence Scanlon, Chairman of CPSC, on ATV Settlement*. Washington, D.C.: Consumer Product Safety Commission.

Ford, GT. 1989. *Final Report on Undercover Investigation of ATV Dealers*. Prepared for U.S. Consumer Product Safety Commission.

Jagger, J. 1990. Seminar presented at Johns Hopkins Injury Prevention Center, Baltimore, Md., April 4.

McKnight, RH. 1984. U.S. Agricultural equipment fatalities, 1975–1981. Doctor of Science thesis, Johns Hopkins University.
Pick, HL. 1987. *ATVs and Children: Perceptual-Motor, Cognitive, and Social Risk Factors.* Prepared for U.S. Consumer Product Safety Commission.
Rivara, FP. 1982. Minibikes: A case study in underregulation, in Bergman, AB. (ed.): *Preventing Childhood Injuries.* Columbus, Ohio: Ross Laboratories.
Rivara, FP. 1985. Fatal and nonfatal farm injuries to children and adolescents in the United States. *Pediatrics* 76(4):567–573.
Swanson, JA, et al. 1987. Accidental farm injuries in children. *Am J Dis Child* 141: 1276–1279.
Tevis, C. 1990. Staying alive . . . The struggle to save farm accident victims. *Successful Farming* March: 37.
Tevis, C, and Finck, C. 1989. We kill too many farm kids, special report. *Successful Farming* Mid-February.
U.S. Department of Transportation. 1988. *Driver License Administration Requirements and Fees–1988.* Publication No. FHWA-PL-88-016. Washington, D.C.: U.S. Dept. of Transportation.
Watson, GS, et al. 1980. The repeal of helmet use laws and increased motorcyclist mortality in the United States: 1975–1978. *Am J Public Health* 70(6):579–585.
Wilkerson, I. 1988. Farms, deadliest workplace, taking the lives of children. *New York Times.* September 26, p. A1.

Additional Sources of Information

Greensher, J. 1988. Non-automotive vehicle injuries in adolescents. *Pediatr Ann* 17(2):114.
National Coalition for Agricultural Safety and Health. 1989. *Agriculture at Risk: A Report to the Nation.* Iowa City: Institute of Agricultural Medicine and Occupational Health, The University of Iowa.

American Academy of Pediatrics (AAP)
141 Northwest Point Boulevard
PO Box 927
Elk Grove Village, IL 60009
312-228-5005
  State Legislation Packet contains model ATV law.

American Society of Agricultural Engineers (ASAE)
2950 Niles Road
St. Joseph, MI 49085
616-429-0300
  Voluntary safety standards for farm equipment.

Farm Safety Association
340 Woodlawn Road West, Suite 22
Guelph, Ontario N1H 7K6
Canada
519-823-5600
  Educational materials, fact sheets, videotapes.

Farm Safety for Just Kids
716 Main Street
PO Box 458
Earlham, IA 50072
515-758-2827
  Educational materials, warning decals, emergency medical treatment handbooks.

The Institute of Agricultural Medicine
and Occupational Health
The University of Iowa
Iowa City, IA 52242
319-335-4415
Educational materials, resource guide, and technical assistance for farm safety efforts.

National Safety Council (NSC)
444 North Michigan Avenue
Chicago, IL 60611
800-621-7619
Educational materials for farm safety.

5

Pedestrians

5.A Facts

Pedestrian injuries are the leading cause of death in children aged 4-8, with the peak at age 6 (see figure 5-1). Each year approximately 1,100 pedestrians aged 0-14 are killed in the traffic environment. In addition, approximately 200 are killed in nontraffic locations such as private driveways, parking lots, and farms, with 1-year-old children at highest risk. Massachusetts rates suggest that emergency rooms treat about 80,000 children annually in the United States who have been injured as pedestrians (Gallagher et al. 1984), many of whom require admission to hospitals.

Because of the tremendous forces involved and the lack of protective structures surrounding the pedestrian, severe multiple injuries are common. Case-fatality rates are very high when head injuries are present and are particularly high for children (Fife 1987). Rates of death and serious injury are about twice as high in boys as in girls, and are especially high in urban and low-income areas. The nontraffic pedestrian death rate, on the other hand, is three times as high in the most rural areas as in urban areas.

Children are struck by cars when they dart into traffic, especially where parked cars obscure them from the view of drivers, cross the street in front of school buses, and walk or crawl near cars in yards and driveways. Injuries are concentrated in the after-school hours from 3:00 to 7:00. During the hour after sunset, when visibility is poor, pedestrian deaths are especially likely.

Prevention requires separating children from vehicular traffic, making it easier for children and cars to see one another, slowing traffic in areas where children are apt to be crossing the street, supervising children until they are old enough to make reliable decisions regarding street crossing, and training those old enough to cross alone.

5.B Developmental Considerations
5.B.1 Infants

Infants are not themselves pedestrians but may be carried or conveyed in a carriage or stroller near motor vehicle traffic. Able-bodied adults, likely to be walking with infants, are not at high risk for pedestrian injury, especially in the daytime. They, and perhaps drivers approaching them, may use particularly cautious behavior. Whatever the reason, infant "pedestrian" injuries are relatively rare.

5.B.2 Toddlers

Toddlers are especially likely to be injured in off-street (nontraffic) pedestrian events. Because their short stature makes them hard to see as they play behind or approach a vehicle from the rear, drivers may back over them.

Toddlers are *absolutely* unreliable around traffic. They cannot be taught appropriate street wisdom. Playing toddlers may follow a toy, animal, or older child into the street. They must be separated from traffic or constantly and closely supervised. Crossing a street with a dawdling toddler can be a frustrating and even frightening experience for an adult, who may react by injuring the child, most often by jerking the child's upraised arm.

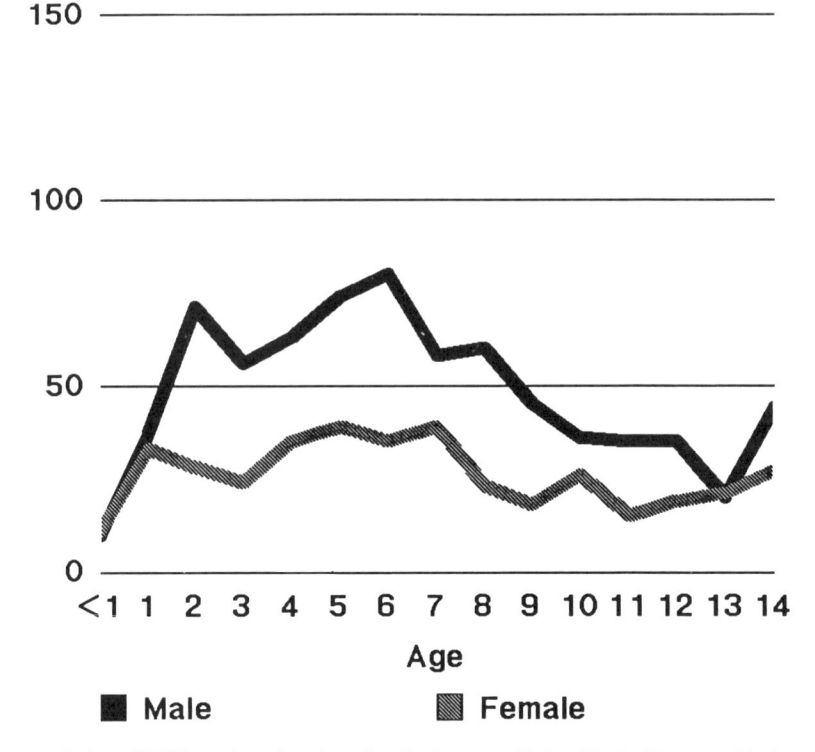

FIGURE 5-1. *Childhood pedestrian deaths by age, U.S., 1986. (Source: National Center for Health Statistics 1988.)*

5.B.3 Preschoolers

Pedestrian injuries increase markedly beginning at about age 4. This increase in the preschool years appears to reflect advances in freedom and mobility that precede children's perceptual maturation and ability to foresee consequences (Pick 1987). Though their pedestrian behavior can be improved with appropriate instruction and training (Preusser and Blomberg 1984; Renaud and Suissa 1989), most children of this age are distractible, variable in their performance of tasks, and slow to react. In addition, they confuse right and left and misjudge distances. Children this size are easily concealed from drivers by parked cars or trucks, bushes, and other roadside structures. Most injuries occur when children run into the street in midblock, often from between parked cars. At times, apparently playing and oblivious, they actually run into the moving vehicle (Campbell 1981). Preschoolers lack the prerequisite abilities and experience for consistent safe crossing—not only in midblock but also at intersections, which are even more complicated because of the need to consider turning vehicles.

5.B.4 Elementary School Ages

Risk of pedestrian injury remains high, especially for males, until at least age 9 or 10, and during the after-school hours. Exposure increases as children walk to and from school and the homes of friends. They may even use the street for recreational activities like roller skating or skateboarding. Perceptual and attention-focusing abilities are still maturing into adolescence and, for some components, beyond. At the age of school entry, children are poorer than adults in detecting objects in the periphery of the visual field and in localizing sound. Many elementary school children still fail to comprehend traffic vocabulary, signals, and patterns, and confuse left and right: only about half of Swedish 8- and 9-year-olds crossed correctly at an intersection when tested in a model traffic situation (Sandels 1970). There is little evidence that adults recognize and compensate for these developmental handicaps that put child pedestrians at increased risk. Parents appear to expect that a schoolchild will cross safely, and drivers expect that a child will yield the right of way.

Physical, as well as neurodevelopmental, growth influences pedestrian injury. The pedestrian's height influences the type, and therefore the severity, of injury. Since most pedestrians are struck by the front of the motor vehicle, not run over, the bodily location of the impact is crucial. While an adult might sustain a broken leg, a short child might suffer a more serious injury of the head or neck.

5.B.5 Young Adolescents

By early adolescence, the highest risk of pedestrian injury during childhood has passed. It is not clear whether this is due entirely to improved street-crossing behavior that results from the cumulative effects of more years of training, more mature abilities, and improved judgment, or whether it is due to a change in exposure as the child begins to spend more transportation time as a bicyclist and a motor vehicle passenger. Circumstances surrounding injury shift: "dart-out" pedestrian injuries are less likely than at earlier ages, but like younger children, young adolescents are injured while playing in the street (Campbell 1981).

5.C Opportunities for Protection

> STRATEGIES FOR PREVENTING INJURIES TO PEDESTRIANS
> (high-priority strategies are indicated by a △)
>
> *Reducing Exposure to Traffic*
> △ Discharge children from cars or buses where they will not need to cross the street.
>   Provide recreational areas separated from vehicles.
>   Design communities to minimize street crossing.
>   Provide safe transportation.
>   Provide sidewalks and create other walkways separated from the traffic flow.
>
> *Increasing Visibility*
> △ Prohibit parking where children are most likely to cross streets.
>   Provide angle parking on one-way streets.
>   Design circular driveways so drivers need not back up.
>   Improve and use mirrors on the fronts of buses.
>   Provide children with reflectors and easily seen clothing.
>
> *Changing the Pedestrian Environment*
> △ Identify and change high-risk sites.
>   Use warning signs and speed bumps.
>   Provide crossings that are safer and easier, such as midblock traffic lights near schools.
>   Pass and/or enforce laws requiring traffic to stop when a school bus is taking on or discharging passengers.
>   Enforce speed limits in areas frequented by children.
>
> *Changing Child Behavior*
>   Train in street-crossing strategies.
>   Teach school-age children not to dart out into the street between intersections.

Changing Adult Behavior
>   Accompany children across streets.
>   Supervise play near streets.
>   Inform adult drivers of special characteristics of child pedestrians.

5.C.1 Schools and Child Care Centers

The efficacy of school-based programs to teach young children safe pedestrian practices has been controversial and may depend on the age of the child. Young children, some have argued, should not be taught how to cross a street but instead should be taught not to cross streets without supervision. Older children should be taught how to watch for oncoming traffic and not to dart into the street between parked cars. Some educational programs have recorded substantial decreases in injury rates for child pedestrians (Preusser and Lund 1988). Age-appropriate educational programs, such as the "Willie Whistle" program developed for the National Highway Traffic Safety Administration (Preusser and Blomberg 1984), should be used with accompanying evaluation.

There is some evidence that the existence of adult crossing guards at busy intersections in school vicinities can reduce the speed of traffic. Schools should provide some form of assistance to children crossing roads at nearby intersections.

Many more children are killed as pedestrians having alighted from school buses than as occupants of school buses. Researchers have found that a swing-out stop arm on a school bus, especially when augmented by a strobe light, reduces the incidence of drivers illegally passing stopped school buses (IIHS 1985; TRB 1989). Schools should use equipment and establish protocols designed to minimize the chances of pedestrian injuries to children approaching and leaving school buses. Partial solutions may include training school bus drivers on the subject of safety at loading and unloading, requiring drivers to escort children across the street, careful planning and annual review of routes and stopping locations to minimize risk to children (e.g., the bus should not be required to back up), and school yard designs that provide safe loading and unloading zones (TRB 1989).

5.C.2 Health Care Providers

Effective anticipatory guidance in the clinical setting to prevent pedestrian injury has not yet been demonstrated. Health care providers might recommend to parents an "age of discretion" at which independent street crossing might be taught and, when skills have been demonstrated, allowed. The specific age will vary with the individual child's abilities and environment. Children younger than 7 should cross only with an adult's assistance. Seven-to nine-year-olds should not cross major streets and should be taught to wait if there is approaching traffic (Rivara et al. 1988). Health care providers also might recommend that parents carefully plan the routes their school-age children use to walk to school or to the homes of friends. Children should be discouraged from walking along roadways but be taught to face traffic (walk on the left) when they must do so. The most powerful role for health care providers is probably in initiating or supporting community coalitions to implement broad programs to prevent pedestrian injury.

5.C.3 Public Agencies

While complete separation of pedestrian and motor vehicle traffic is the ideal, strategies that decrease through traffic and the speed of traffic in residential areas can decrease pedestrian injury. Such strategies include creating culs-de-sac, narrow and one-way streets as well as building in bumps and obstacles. Demonstrations of "environmental control" in Europe have markedly decreased childhood injury (Brownfield 1980; Kane 1985). Parking patterns along the street probably influence the likelihood of pedestrian injury because they may allow access to the street between intersections or limit the driver's view of children about to enter the street. Diagonal parking and crossing barriers attached to parking meters may reduce injury (Berger 1975). This issue deserves more study. Crosswalk markings may actually contribute to injury by falsely assuring pedestrians of safety without deterring drivers. Their efficacy needs study.

Developers and planners have an ideal opportunity to ensure child pedestrian safety when laying out new communities. Separating pedestrians from traffic and ensuring walking routes to schools and parks that do not force children to cross major roads are two examples. Transportation or traffic safety agencies can study the geography of pedestrian injury within a community to pinpoint locations where special action is needed—a light or obstacle to slow down traffic, relocation of bus stops to the far side of intersections, the banning of right turns on red, improved roadway lighting, a fence that precludes crossing except at a controlled intersection, a convenient pedestrian walkway, or a crossing guard, to name a number of strategies that might be considered. In particular, roadways in the vicinity of schools and play areas should be monitored to determine whether speed or traffic flow should be modified for the protection of children.

5.C.4 Legislators and Regulators

Several legislative interventions are likely to reduce the incidence of childhood pedestrian injuries. Zoning laws and regulations at the local level can require sidewalks and a "buffer zone" between vehicular traffic and pedestrian walkways. Particular attention might be paid to areas frequented by children (e.g., school and playground areas) and to areas of high vehicular density. Speed in these areas can be limited, and visibility unobstructed by shrubs, fences, and other structures.

States and/or localities can consider strategies to increase the effectiveness of laws requiring motorists to stop when approaching or following a school bus stopped to accept or discharge passengers. Such laws now are frequently ignored (TRB 1989). Supplementing the basic legislation with other measures, such as those enabling bus drivers to report violators, is one possibility. School buses themselves can be regulated so that lights and/ or other mechanisms unequivocally warn motorists to stop. Strobe lights on stop-signal arms are likely to improve current signal systems. Local lawmakers can specify safety features for school buses used in their area. For instance, crossing-control arms that force children to walk widely around the bus keep them in the driver's view.

The use of other vehicles, such as ice cream trucks, can be regulated to avoid "Pied Piper injuries," which occur when children are attracted into the street. Requiring vendors to display warning signals and passing drivers to stop and yield to pedestrians may be a partial solution (Blomberg et al. 1978).

Permitting drivers to turn right following a stop at a red light increases the number of pedestrian injuries (Zador et al. 1982; Preusser et al. 1982). If such laws are to be preserved because other considerations, such as traffic flow and air pollution, take precedence over pedestrian safety, drivers and pedestrians should be educated about the risks involved.

At the federal level, regulators might explore the possibility of modifying the front of motor vehicles to reduce the severity of injury to a child who is struck. The fact that children are struck and killed by their own school buses suggests that cross-view mirrors currently required by Federal Motor Vehicle Safety Standards may not afford drivers an adequate view of small children in front of the school bus. Modifications to the standard should be considered (TRB 1989).

5.C.5 Law Enforcement Professionals

Strict enforcement of speed limits in school areas and at times children are going to and from school is recommended. Similarly, the presence of law enforcement officers on streets at events frequented by children may reduce the likelihood of pedestrian injuries. Driver intoxication should be considered in pedestrian as well as vehicle crashes.

Motorists meeting or overtaking a school bus stopped to board or discharge passengers (with warning lights flashing) are required to stop by transportation codes in many areas. This measure decreases the likelihood that a child will step into the path of a passing vehicle. Violations are common, but frequently police are not present to observe and apprehend the violator. Transportation codes can be amended to permit police to issue a warning letter to the registered owner of any vehicle observed by a school bus operator to violate such laws. Police and school officials can cooperate with school bus contractors to educate the public about school bus laws and to encourage school bus operators to report violators to the police. Law enforcement professionals can exert a strong and influential presence in schools and in community coalitions to decrease pedestrian injury.

5.C.6 Voluntary Organizations

Organizations that use old school buses for transporting children should retrofit the buses with up-to-date safety equipment (mirrors, swing-out signal arms, crossing arms, etc.) or use new buses (TRB 1989). Adult supervision of child pedestrians on group outings should be rigorous, and routes should be carefully planned to avoid traffic.

A program to increase child-pedestrian visibility by distributing reflective dots for clothing has been related to a reduced child pedestrian death rate (Kane 1985). Leg lamps or flashlights may increase driver recognition of pedestrians even more. Organizations might promote these strategies, at the same time taking care not to encourage children to walk near or across roadways after dark.

Pedestrian safety clubs have been related to reductions of pedestrian injuries in Europe (Kane 1985). Organizations in the United States might participate in similar clubs with careful evaluation. Providing play spaces that are divided from traffic but not isolated, so that children will use them, is an attractive concept.

5.C.7 Designers, Architects, Builders, and Engineers

The front end of the motor vehicle most often hits the pedestrian. Design modifications that take into account children's short stature (changes in bumper and hood design) might decrease the severity of injury.

Pedestrians are more visible at night when their clothing includes reflective materials. Although such materials might be a welcome addition in outerwear and might be used to make lightweight safety vests for summer use, probably only a small reduction in childhood pedestrian injuries would result, since most of these injuries do not occur at night. Lights are even more readily recognized by drivers than reflective materials. Special "walking lights" might be designed.

A number of structural initiatives that might reduce childhood pedestrian injuries have been mentioned in other sections. These include planning for safe school bus loading and unloading areas when school yards are designed, planning safe walking routes to schools and parks when new developments or communities are laid out, instituting traffic- and parking-control initiatives, providing play areas as enticing as but safer than streets, erecting barriers that prevent pedestrian egress into high-speed traffic, and providing convenient pedestrian walkways over or under motor vehicle traffic. Signal systems for school buses are confusing and ignored by many motorists. Designs that have been shown to improve compliance by motorists include fold-out stop-signal arms, especially when enhanced by strobe lights (TRB 1989). Modifications that make the child visible to the bus driver while approaching or leaving the bus are needed. These might include enhanced mirror systems, other types of sensors, and barriers attached to the bus that force the child far enough away from the bus to be seen. In addition, much exciting work remains to be done in the design of traffic and pedestrian control signals so that children understand them. Even basic pictographs now used are misunderstood by children.

5.C.8 Business and Industry

Businesses can prevent child pedestrian injuries in their environs and parking lots by providing structural separation of pedestrians and motor traffic wherever possible. Traffic lights, crossing guards, and signs that children can understand are other measures that might be implemented to protect child pedestrians. Special attention should be paid to pedestrian risks from trucks serving the business.

Reflective outerwear for children may provide protection from injuries by increasing their visibility to the drivers of motor vehicles. The marketing of poorly reflective look-alike designs may confuse consumers who assume they are getting protection which is not provided.

5.C.9 Mass Media

Preventing pedestrian injury is particularly frustrating because few strategies for automatically protecting children are known. The best protection is afforded by environmental designs that separate children from motor vehicle traffic. Once streets and buildings are in place, however, this is difficult, so preventing pedestrian injury relies heavily on the behavior of children as they play near and cross streets, the supervision of parents and other adults, and the behavior of those who drive. The mass media can help to shape the behavior of children and adults by carefully crafted messages. Crossing behavior has been improved and injuries decreased for children in the high-risk age-group by campaigns that included media exhortations to stop at the curb and look left, right, left before entering the street (Preusser and Blomberg 1984). Specific messages highlighting child pedestrians designed to change behavior of parents and drivers might also be effective.

Reporters can help to prevent future pedestrian injuries by looking for patterns. If injury has occurred repeatedly at a particular intersection or in front of a particular school or business, highlighting the pattern in news coverage can prompt remedial action such as slowing or diverting traffic, or building a pedestrian walkway.

References

American Automobile Association. 1982. *The Young Pedestrian.* Pedestrian Safety Program Series No. 3. Falls Church, Va.: American Automobile Association.

Berger, WG. 1975. *Urban Pedestrian Accident Countermeasures Experimental Evaluation.* Vol. 1, *Behavioral Evaluation Studies.* (DOT HS-801 346). Washington, D.C.: National Highway Traffic Safety Administration.

Blomberg, RD, et al. 1978. *Experimental Field Test of the Model Ice Cream Truck Ordinance in Detroit.* (Publication No. PB-283419). Springfield, Va.: National Technical Information Service.

Brownfield, DJ. 1980. Environmental areas—interim report on a before-and-after accident study. *Traffic Engineering and Control* 21:278-282.

Campbell, BJ. 1981. *The Young Child in Pedestrian Accidents.* Chapel Hill, N.C.: University of North Carolina Highway Safety Research Center.

Fife, D. 1987. Time from injury to death (survival time) among fatally injured pedestrians. *Injury* 18:315-318.

Gallagher, S, et al. 1984. The incidence of injuries among 87,000 Massachusetts children and adolescents: Results of the 1980-81 Statewide Childhood Injury Prevention Program surveillance system. *Am J Public Health* 74(12):1340-1347.

Insurance Institute for Highway Safety. 1985. Two Texas studies probe illegal passing of school buses. *The Highway Loss Reduction Status Report*—Special Issue, School Buses and Seat Belts 20(5):9.

Kane, DN. 1985. *Environmental Hazards to Young Children.* Phoenix: Oryx Press.

National Center for Health Statistics. 1988. *Vital Statistics of the United States, 1986.* Vol. 2, Mortality, pt. A. Dept. of Health and Human Services publication No. (PHS) 88-1122. Washington, D.C.: U.S. Government Printing Office.

Preusser, DF, and Blomberg, RD. 1984. Reducing child pedestrian accidents through public education. *Journal of Safety Research* 15(2):47-56.

Preusser, DF, and Lund, AK. 1988. And Keep on Looking: A film to reduce pedestrian crashes among 9 to 12 year olds. *Journal of Safety Research* 19(4):177-185.

Preusser, DF, et al. 1982. The effect of right-turn-on-red on pedestrian and bicyclist accidents. *Journal of Safety Research* 13(2):45-55.

Renaud, L, and Suissa, S. 1989. Evaluation of the efficacy of simulation games in traffic safety education of kindergarten children. *Am J Public Health* 79(3):307-309.

Rivara, FP, et al. 1988. *Strategies for Preventing Child Pedestrian Injuries,* position paper. Seattle: Harborview Injury Prevention and Research Center.

Sandels, S. 1970. Young children in traffic. *Br J Educ Psychol* 40(2):111-116.

Transportation Research Board. 1989. *Improving School Bus Safety.* Special Report 222. Washington, D.C.: Transportation Research Board.

Zador, P, et al. 1982. Adoption of right turn on red: Effects on crashes at signalized intersections. *Accid Anal Prev* 14(3):219-234.

Additional Sources of Information

American Automobile Association (AAA)
Foundation for Traffic Safety
1730 M Street, NW
Suite 401
Washington, DC 20036
202-775-1456
 (or local AAA clubs)
 Educational materials and reports.

Harborview Injury Prevention and Research Center
325 Ninth Avenue, ZX-10
Seattle, WA 98104
206-223-3158
 Educational materials, including the Wary Walker Pedestrian Education Program.

National Highway Traffic Safety Administration (NHTSA)
Routing Symbol NTS-23
400 7th Street, SW
Washington, DC 20590
202-366-2761
 Educational materials, including the Willie Whistle Program, various reports, such as *Pedestrian Safety Bibliography: Selected Current Research and Studies*, which includes reports on model legislation.

Royal Society for the Prevention of Accidents (RoSPA)
Cannon House, The Priory Queensway
Birmingham, B4 6BS
UK
 Educational materials, including the Tufty Club, preschool pedestrian educational program.

Society of Automotive Engineers (SAE)
400 Commonwealth Drive
Warrendale, PA 15096
412-776-4841
 Research reports.

Transport and Road Research Laboratory (TRRL)
Department of Transport
Old Wokingham Road
Crowthorne Berkshire RG11 6AU
UK
 Research reports on roadway design and pedestrian safety.

Transportation Research Board (TRB)
National Research Council
2101 Constitution Avenue, NW
Washington, DC 20418
202-334-2933
 Research reports.

6
Bicyclists

6.A Facts

Bicycles are associated with more childhood injuries than any other consumer product except the automobile. Each year about 400 children under 15 years old are killed in the United States while riding bicycles and almost 400,000 require emergency room treatment.

Children aged 6–15 have high death rates from bicycle-related injuries (see figure 6–1), although this is an age-group for which injury death rates as a whole are *lower* than for other ages. Death rates are four times as high for males as for females. Four deaths out of five result from head injuries, and about 90% involve collisions with motor vehicles.

The head and neck sustain the primary injury in about one-third of children treated (Selbst et al. 1987). Other serious injuries include abdominal injuries from contact with handlebars, foot injuries from entanglement in bicycle spokes, and genital injuries from falling or sliding onto the top bar of the bicycle frame.

The most serious bicyclist injuries result from bicycle–motor vehicle collisions, but the majority of injuries involve falls and collisions with stationary objects, other bicycles, or pedestrians. The marked increase in injuries in spring and summer offers opportunities for well-timed preventive programs.

Circumstances that contribute to bicyclist injuries include performing stunts or speeding, riding double, road hazards (e.g., loose gravel, road grates that catch wheels), loss of control on downhill slopes, product failure, poor bicycle maintenance, and bicyclist error or inexperience. Bike–car collisions frequently involve the bicyclist entering a road without stopping, riding against traffic, running a stop sign, turning without warning, or riding at night. The contribution of the motor vehicle operator has not been adequately explored, but the difficulty of seeing cyclists in twilight or darkness indicates the need for reflective or light-colored clothing, as well as adequate lights and reflectors on bicycles.

The importance of brain injury as a cause of death or permanent disability means that cyclists of all ages should wear helmets meeting the standards set by the Snell Memorial Foundation and/or the American National Standards Institute (ANSI). (Both organizations test helmets in the same way,

Number of Deaths

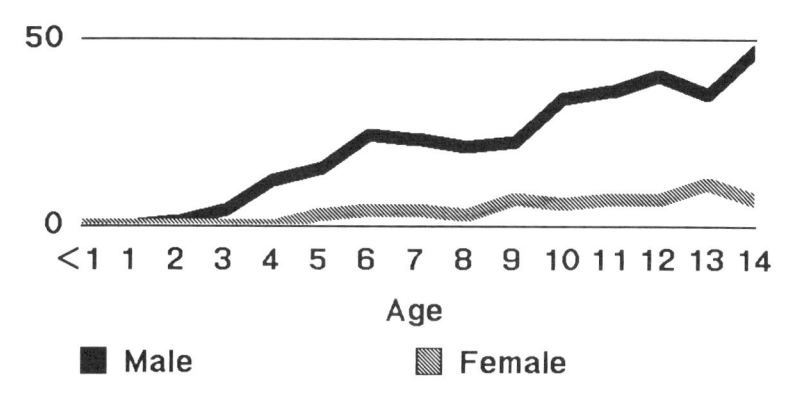

[Chart showing number of deaths by age (<1 to 14) for Male and Female]

FIGURE 6-1. *Childhood bicyclist deaths by age, U.S., 1986. (Source: National Center for Health Statistics 1988.)*

by determining deceleration inside a helmeted head form dropped onto metal anvils a number of times. The ANSI standard is a consensus standard, however, which means that manufacturers and other interested parties develop and approve the standard. Consensus standards are generally less rigid than independent standards. See additional sources of information.) Any helmet struck in a crash or fall should be replaced.

Recent research indicates that helmets reduce head injury in bicyclists by as much as 85% (Thompson et al. 1989). Helmet use is now required for U.S. Cycling Federation racers and is increasing among older cyclists. Young children, on the other hand, must depend on their parents to purchase helmets for them, and are the group least often protected and at greatest risk for bicycle-related head injuries. In Victoria, Australia, an intensive campaign that included carefully designed educational components and rebates for people who purchased helmets increased helmet use by primary school children from 5 to 39% in a two-year period (Wood and Milne 1988). Multifaceted helmet campaigns in the United States have also met with modest success (Bergman et al. 1990).

6.B Developmental Considerations

6.B.1 and 6.B.2 Infants and Toddlers

Infants and toddlers may be injured as bicycle passengers when they fall from or with the bike, when their dangling extremities are caught in the spokes of the wheels, or when the bicycle collides with a vehicle or another object. Transporting an infant or toddler as a passenger provides an additional challenge for the bicycle operator, because the child's weight and movement may contribute to loss of control of the vehicle and may increase stopping distance. This added challenge may exceed the competence of even normally proficient adult cyclists; it certainly is likely to do so for younger, less experienced, and less powerful cyclists. Carrying passengers on a bicycle under even the best of circumstances should be discouraged. Children should not be allowed to transport any passenger, including infants and toddlers. Carrier seats and helmets, however, have been designed specifically to protect children of this age-group, for adults who choose to cycle with young child passengers (see section 6.C.2).

6.B.3 Preschoolers

During the preschool years most children become cyclists themselves, and 90% can pedal a three-wheeled vehicle by 3 years of age. As children approach school age, their interest in two-wheeled vehicles increases. They may ride as a passenger with an older child. This is particularly hazardous behavior when the driver is young, as noted earlier.

In one Vermont city, two-thirds of children in kindergarten owned two-wheelers (Waller 1971), and the average age of learning to ride was between 5 and 6 years. Riding a bicycle requires sophisticated motor skills—young learners wobble and fall frequently. In addition to the challenge of balancing, they must master the particularly difficult tasks of starting and stopping without falling. Like a toddler learning to walk, a young cyclist may fall due to slight bumps, turns, and distractions. The beginning rider is unpredictable and preoccupied with managing the bike itself; therefore hazards of the riding environment must be minimized. This argues for strictly discouraging young riders from transporting passengers and riding near traffic.

6.B.4 Elementary School Ages

In the citywide study mentioned earlier, 80 to 90% of elementary schoolchildren owned bikes. About one-third of the third- and fourth-grade boys were already riding after dark.

Children are able to ride a two-wheeled bicycle long before they have the judgment to do so safely in traffic. Specifically, they are only marginally able to judge speeds and distances, which puts them in jeopardy when riding on streets with motor vehicles. Peer pressure takes on increasing importance during this period, with the peak years for conformity to peers coming at ages 11 to 13. Children are particularly likely to reject protective gear, bike designs, or riding behaviors not sanctioned by their peer group.

Although children in this age-group do not grow as quickly as infants and adolescents, they grow rapidly enough that they often may be riding bicycles that are too small for them or have been purchased too large so they can be used for a number of years. Bicycles of the wrong size are said to contribute to control difficulties for the rider and therefore to injury. The American Academy of Pediatrics includes the following in its guidelines for choosing a bicycle (AAP 1987):

1. The child should be able to place the balls of both feet on the ground when sitting on the seat with the hands on the handlebars.
2. Straddling the center bar should be possible with both feet flat on the ground; there should be about 1 inch clearance between the crotch and the bar.
3. The handlebars should be within easy reach.

6.B.5 Young Adolescents

For many preteens the bicycle is the major form of independent transportation. As adolescence progresses, bicycles serve as a car substitute. Friendship circles widen, outside activities and jobs become more common, and parental supervision decreases. Neighborhood boundaries become less relevant in adolescence, and more of the rider's time may be spent outside familiar territory. Adolescents are likely to ride bicycles farther from home than before, on roadways shared by motor vehicles, and after dark. Peer pressure to conform to group standards, mentioned earlier, is very important.

6.C Opportunities for Protection

STRATEGIES FOR PREVENTING INJURIES TO BICYCLISTS
(high-priority strategies are indicated by a △)

Increasing Helmet Use

△ Pass legislation requiring helmet use.
△ Promote helmet use.
△ Make helmets inexpensive and easy to find.
△ Make helmets comfortable and appealing.

Increasing Visibility

△ Provide reflective clothing.
  Require bicycle lights and reflectors for cycling after dark.
  Encourage use of leg lamps and reflective clothing.

Changing the Bicycling Environment

△ Separate bicyclists from motor vehicle traffic with bikeways and physical barriers.

Improve the riding surface.

Changing Equipment

Delete top bar of boy's bicycle design.
Provide spoke covers or solid wheel design.
Provide chain covers.

Changing Child Behavior

Teach traffic laws.
Provide bicycle proficiency training.
Discourage excessive speed, stunt riding, and riding double.

6.C.1 Schools and Child Care Centers

Regulation by schools of the use of bicycles on school grounds has proven effective. In Victoria, Australia, for example, some schools required that all children who ride their bikes to school wear helmets; the schools purchased approved helmets in bulk and offered them to parents at a reduced price. Rates of bicycle helmet use among children increased, and head injuries among bicycle crash victims decreased, without apparent negative effects (Wood and Milne 1988). Schools that establish a compulsory helmet rule should be certain that the helmets required are those that meet established safety standards (the Snell and/or the ANSI standards discussed in section 6.A), that secure storage space for helmets is available to the children, and that there is enforcement of the rule. At least one helmet manufacturer provides discount coupons to schools and other groups. Local bike shops may also offer helmet discounts to schools.

In accord with the traditional educational role of schools, bicycle safety and injury prevention can be incorporated into the school curriculum (see additional sources of information). Many existing educational programs use someone from outside the school, such as a police officer, to present the information. These programs, however, may not adequately stress the use of bike helmets, which is of utmost importance in reducing the most serious injuries to bicycling children. Children should be taught that the rules of the road apply to bicyclists. They should be made aware of the most frequently occurring errors, such as failing to signal and/or look behind when turning or changing lanes, failing to ride in single file, and riding on the wrong side of the road (Dewar 1978), and should be trained in the correct riding techniques on bikes when possible. Instructors should teach children to perform regular upkeep and safety checks on their bikes.

Additional school-related activities mentioned as a means of focusing attention on bike safety are contests among schools for the most helmet wearers; helmet-decorating workshops, during which children decorate their helmets with stickers or reflective tape; bike rodeos; and bike inspection and registration programs. These measures are unevaluated interventions that should be used only to supplement the measures listed above, not to replace them, and should be carefully planned to ensure that they address the issues most likely to prevent injury—wearing helmets, avoiding traffic, and riding predictably.

6.C.2 Health Care Providers

Few pediatricians and family physicians have routinely included bicycling in patient education (Weiss and Duncan 1986), although it is one of the leading causes of childhood morbidity and mortality. A physician's resource manual on bicycle safety is now available from the American Academy of Pediatrics (see additional sources of information). When targeting anticipatory guidance on the subject of bicycle injury, the following points should be kept in mind:

1. School-age males are the group at highest risk of death.
2. Children who do not own bicycles may not be confidently exempted; apparently, children quite commonly share bikes with friends.
3. Children too young to operate bicycles may be passengers on bicycles ridden by older children or adults.
4. Children who ride on the street—for instance, to and from school— are at additional risk because the bulk of serious injuries are sustained in crashes with motor vehicles.

Above all else, children should be encouraged to wear a helmet while riding; information about helmets and helmet discount coupons from bike shops or manufacturers may be provided to the children and the parents. Behaviors that have been related to injury, such as riding double and stunt riding, may be discouraged during health education. Because crashes with motor vehicles result in the most serious injuries, parents should be encouraged to delay street riding until the child has had appropriate training in traffic regulations and experience and is at least 9 years old. Even then, routes should avoid heavy traffic at least until the child is a licensed driver. Night riding should be prohibited or discouraged; if undertaken by older children, functioning head- and taillights are necessary, and leg lamps and reflective clothing may be helpful.

Loss of control is cited as a causal factor in a large proportion of bicycling injuries and may be exacerbated by bicycles that are too large for the child. Parents may be advised of the additional risk that may accrue when bicycles are bought large for children to "grow into" (see section 6.B.4 for size guidance). The likelihood of injury is also increased when the bicycle is in poor repair (loose pedals, loose steering column, malfunctioning brakes, etc.). Regular inspections by the parent are in order.

Because of the inherent risks, parents should be discouraged from transporting children as passengers on bicycles. If parents are not dissuaded, the recommendations of the American Academy of Pediatrics should be provided. They are, in summary, the following (AAP 1987):

1. Children younger than 6 months should not be carried.
2. Children between 6 and 12 months should be carried in a backpack carrier or bicycle cart.
3. Children 12 months or older can be belted into a properly installed and maintained seat that protects the hands and feet from spokes and minimizes the risk of falling. In addition, traffic should be avoided and the parent and child should wear helmets.

A final topic in a discussion of bicycle safety could be to encourage the use of bicycles instead of motorized vehicles for children (motorbikes, ATVs). Health care providers should vehemently discourage purchase of motorized vehicles for children because of their excessive injury rates (see chapter 4, Users of Other Motor Vehicles).

In addition to providing guidance to individual families, health care providers may act together through their professional organizations to bring bicycle injuries to public attention and to promote prevention by providing news releases to the media and sponsoring public-service announcements. A video announcement suggesting the use of helmets to which the name of a sponsoring group can be added is available from the Harborview Injury Prevention Center, for instance (see additional sources of information). If no bicycle training is available in the community, health care providers can act as individuals or groups to be certain it is offered, and can help to sustain it by referring patients.

6.C.3 Public Agencies

Public agencies, such as community planners and departments of transportation, can be instrumental in designing and maintaining a bicycling environment to maximize safety. Bicyclists have the same rights and responsibilities as motor vehicle operators in almost all states. Transportation or highway departments are responsible for providing roads that are safe for bicyclists. For example, storm drains in roadways used by bicyclists should have grates that are perpendicular to the flow of traffic, to prevent bicycle wheels from getting caught in the grates. Resources are available for designing bike paths and bicycle-compatible roadways (see additional sources of information).

One study (McFarlane et al. 1982) found that "the condition of the road surface was the most common factor contributing to bicycle trauma." Road surfaces and edges should be free of loose gravel (Burgess and Burden 1977) and roads should be well lighted. Potholes, tree limbs, crumbling edges, and other obstacles on the roadway or shoulder can be hazardous to bicyclists.

One method of reducing the number and severity of injuries to child bicyclists is to separate them from the flow of car and truck traffic. Public agencies can effect this by creating cycling areas and paths that are not on the shoulders of streets and highways. If designated bicycle paths are not feasible, physical barriers can be used to separate bicycle traffic from other traffic, motor vehicle traffic can be rerouted, and/or speeds can be reduced on roads that are designated bike routes (Friede et al. 1985).

Many adults are not alert to bicyclists in traffic, especially child bicyclists. Research has shown that many adults overestimate children's ability to ride in traffic (Sandels 1974) and knowledge of traffic rules. Motor vehicle administrations should include material on the rights and limitations of child cyclists in their driving handbooks and license tests.

The Road Traffic Authority of Victoria, Australia, conducted the successful campaign to promote bicycle helmet use and reduce head injuries to bicyclists mentioned earlier (see sections 6.A and 6.C.1). Helmet-promotion campaigns could be sponsored in the United States by any combination of agencies.

6.C.4 Legislators and Regulators

Bicyclists are protected by legislative measures that protect all users of the highways, such as laws addressing drunk driving. In addition, some laws protect bicyclists specifically. Legally, bicyclists, including children, are obligated to obey the same rules of the road as cars; for example, they must stop for red lights and travel in the proper direction on one-way streets.

Vehicle and traffic codes should be reviewed with bicycle safety in mind to determine whether amendments might be required to provide maximum protection for bicyclists. State laws should at least conform to the Uniform Vehicle Code, and may offer additional protection. The state of California, for example, amended its vehicle code in 1986 to prohibit riding double and to provide for the safety of bicycle passengers who are 4 years old or younger, or who weigh 40 pounds or less (California General Assembly 1986). These passengers may ride only in a seat that retains them in place and protects them from the bicycle's moving parts and must wear a helmet that meets ANSI or Snell standards. A first violation of the helmet provision is dismissed if the violator produces proof that a proper helmet has been purchased. Legislation requiring helmet use has been enacted in one Maryland county and is highly recommended.

Lamps, reflectors, and reflective strips on bikes, bicyclists, or their clothing can be expected to increase the bicyclist's visibility to motorists and therefore decrease injury. Tests suggest that leg lamps, for instance, would allow earlier detection and recognition than the reflectors required by present regulations (Blomberg et al. 1986). While bicycling or walking on the roadway at night cannot be recommended as safe under any conditions, lamps appear to enhance the conspicuity of both bicyclists and pedestrians more than other reasonably priced alternatives. Legislation can ensure that bicyclists use lights in addition to reflectors. The Massachusetts legislature, for example, passed a law requiring cyclists riding at night to display a front white lamp visible for 500 feet and a rear red reflector or lamp visible for 600 feet (SCIPP 1983). Bicycles themselves are regulated for product safety by the U.S. Consumer Product Safety Commission. Requirements for braking systems, steering systems, pedals, the drive chain, protective guards, tires, wheels and wheel hubs, front fork, fork and frame assembly, seat, reflectors, instructions, and labeling are included (CPSC 1988). Regulations should be enhanced aggressively as new data indicate opportunities for additional safeguards. A possible innovation would be to require purchase of a helmet with each bicycle (Dannenberg 1989).

No mandatory standards exist for bicycle helmets. Voluntary standards are discussed in sections 6.A. and 6.C.7.

6.C.5 Law Enforcement Professionals

Although most states require that bicyclists obey the state traffic laws, enforcement is uncommon. Police programs on the local level should make bicyclists aware of the laws that apply to them and the safety reasons for obeying. Officers should also enforce bicyclists' rights to the road, stopping motorists seen violating those rights or driving in a manner unsafe to bicyclists.

Selective enforcement of the laws, with warnings issued to childhood violators and their parents, may enhance safe bicycling. Some police departments have tried a "bike violators' seminar" for child bicyclists who violate traffic laws, combining enforcement with an educational program. This approach was found to reduce the number of bicycle accidents by 30% or more in 7 of 11 Minnesota communities initiating the program (Friede et al. 1985). The Minnesota program takes advantage of summer vacationing high school and college students, who are trained to issue citations and run the seminars, to augment police personnel who cannot be spared to devote full-time attention to the program (see additional sources of information).

6.C.6 Voluntary Organizations

Voluntary organizations can direct their injury-prevention efforts toward assuring safe practices on the part of bicycle riders and motorists sharing roadways and toward providing a safe riding environment.

Many strategies and materials are available to groups wishing to promote bicycle helmet use (see additional sources of information). An information campaign can be coordinated to involve the local media, businesses, and schools. Many local bike shops and at least one manufacturer make helmet discount coupons available to nonprofit groups. A few community-based bicycle-safety campaigns have been evaluated (DiGuiseppi et al. 1989), and community-based health promotion efforts in other areas (seat belts, for example) have shown some efficacy. A "bike month," during which prevention of bicycle injury becomes a community-wide theme, could be organized. Helmet-decorating workshops have been suggested, but not tested, as a way to make wearing helmets more attractive (Williams 1984) and could be part of such a campaign, as could competitions among schools or other contests. Helmeted racers could be used as role models.

Voluntary organizations can work with law enforcement agencies to be certain that traffic regulations that apply to bicyclists become common knowledge and are enforced. In addition, communities should make bicycle proficiency courses available and accessible to children and parents. In some areas this may be provided through the school system (see section 6.C.1), with the advantage that nearly all children will be reached. Schools may not be able to devote sufficient time to the issue, however, or to provide "on-the-bike" training. Complementary courses can be offered under other auspices. Age-appropriate course content has been designed by several groups. It is highly desirable that bicycle proficiency be achieved before the ages at which street riding is common (8 or 9 years old) and that it be reinforced periodically.

Although it is acknowledged that older children do and will continue to ride on roadways, voluntary organizations can work in their communities to provide attractive alternatives such as bike courses in parks for recreational riding. Ideally, these paths would be free of pedestrians who might be struck by the bicyclists. Many groups are working with the Rails-to-Trails Conservancy to convert abandoned railroad corridors to bicycle and hiking paths. Some paths have two parallel trails—a paved trail for bicycles, strollers, etc., and a dirt trail for joggers and horses. When only one trail is possible, it should be 8 feet wide to allow safe passing of pedestrians by bicycles.

6.C.7 Designers, Architects, Builders, and Engineers

Opportunities for decreasing bicycle injuries include modification of existing protective gear and development of new protective gear to be worn by the rider; modification of the bicycle; improvement of the riding surface; and modification of structures which hit or are hit by cyclists.

Helmets offer the best-known protection against the most serious consequence of bicycle crashes and falls—head injury. Helmet design innovations can decrease injuries in two ways: by improving protection afforded when the helmet is worn and by making helmets more acceptable and therefore more likely to be worn.

Helmet design issues still being debated include whether a hard or soft outer shell is preferable, the quality of protection at the sides of the head, and the security of the buckle and appropriate performance standards. One problem with current voluntary standards is that they do not address the issue of roll-off resistance (the helmet's ability to stay on the wearer's head during a crash) (Consumer Reports 1990). Experts do not know through how many years of use a helmet retains its maximum protective properties. Manufacturers usually recommend replacement after 5 years. Performance information is needed. In addition to limiting head injury in crashes and falls, helmets should be well ventilated and therefore not too hot, comfortable, easy to put on, light, inexpensive, and easy to maintain. They should not obstruct vision or interfere with eyeglasses, and should keep sweat from flowing into the eyes (WABA 1979). Children are more likely to wear helmets if they consider them fashionable, so a child's changing tastes as well as increasing head size must be considered by designers.

Several bicycle design features have been implicated in injury-related events: abdominal injuries may follow a fall onto the handlebars (Sparnon and Ford 1986); injury to the genitalia or perineum is associated with a straddle fall onto the top bar of the boy's bicycle design; clothing or extremities may become entangled in the wheel spokes, causing direct injury or loss of control; fingers have been amputated in chains. These features can be modified or eliminated. Bicycles for children with solid wheel design are now available, for example. It has been suggested that banana-seat designs contribute to two behaviors commonly associated with injury—stunt riding and riding double. Bicycle designers might eliminate this feature. Stability comparisons among children's bicycle designs would be useful.

Failure of most moving or adjustable parts of bicycles has been implicated in injury events. Shoes slip on pedals or pedals come off, handlebars loosen unexpectedly, seats come loose during riding, chains slip. New designs that make such parts less likely to fail and easier to maintain than current designs should decrease injury.

Reflective cycling clothing has been suggested for nighttime wear. Such clothing should not be available in sizes so small that nighttime riding by young children is implicitly condoned. Tests suggest that leg lamps may make bicyclists more conspicuous than other measures (Blomberg et al. 1986). In general, devices intended to make the bicyclist more visible or noticeable, such as lights, reflectors, horns, bells, are often mentioned as important safety features, although most have received little study and, if effective, might be improved. Spacer flags projecting perpendicular to the bike have been used in Scandinavia and Great Britain but not evaluated in the United States as a way to warn motorists to allow cyclists more space (Watts 1983). If they are found to be effective, they must be designed to be durable without contributing to injury in a fall or crash.

Certain features of roadways which have been primarily designed for motor vehicles may be hazards for bicyclists. Such features include speed bumps, uneven pavement surfaces, and drainage grates. In designing surfacing for bikeways, consideration should be given to the likelihood of injury when a cyclist falls on it, in addition to such features as durability and maintenance costs (see additional sources of information).

Lastly, injuries to bicyclists may be caused by the design of vehicles with which they share the roadways; for example, deaths have resulted when the extended rearview mirror of a van or truck struck a cyclist riding along the roadway. Creative solutions to this problem provide an opportunity to prevent rare but severe injury.

6.C.8 Business and Industry

Those who distribute and market bicycles could make a major contribution to injury prevention by vigorously promoting helmet sales. Purchasers of bicycles should be encouraged to purchase helmets. This might be done by showing helmeted riders in ads, placing helmets next to bicycles for sale, reducing helmet prices, giving the purchaser of a new bicycle a discount on a helmet, and recommending a helmet in all printed material and verbal sales interactions. Manufacturers could agree to include a helmet with every bike purchase (Dannenberg 1989). Helmet manufacturers might provide discount coupons to schools and other groups. At least one manufacturer offers free replacements for any of its helmets that have been in a crash when returned with a crash story.

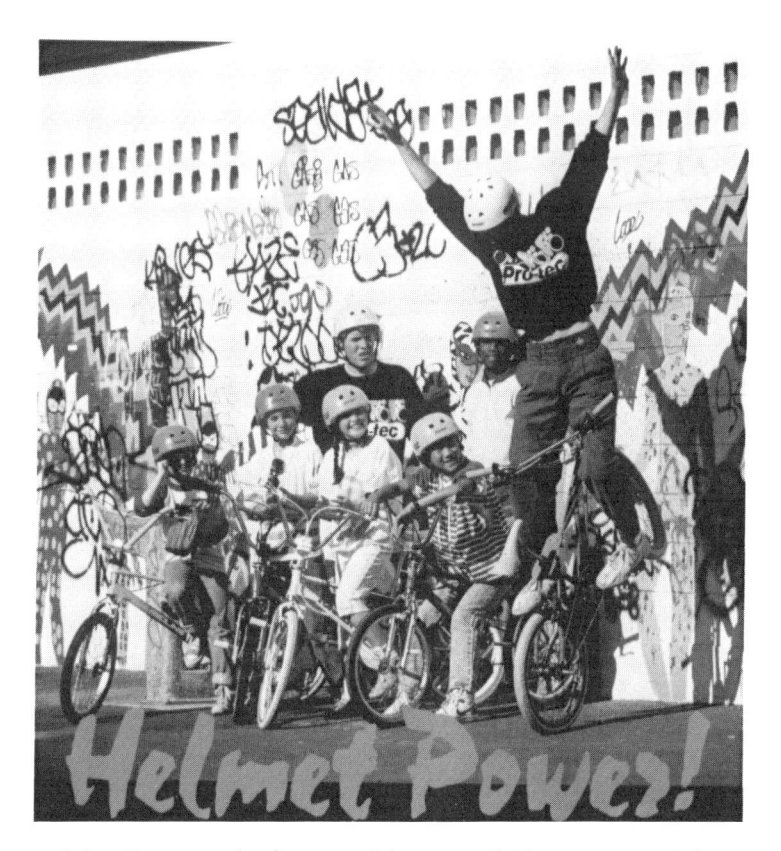

FIGURE 6-2. *Posters and other materials are available to promote helmet acceptance. (Copyright 1988 by Harborview Injury Prevention and Research Center. Reprinted by permission.)*

Sales personnel should be familiar with the rationale for helmets, be able to discuss their attributes, and be able to help with fitting. Some local bike shops offer helmet discounts and educational presentations.

6.C.9 Mass Media

The single most important message to be brought to the public's attention is that bicyclists should wear helmets (see figure 6-2). Public-service announcements have been an important component of initial successful efforts to promote helmet wearing (Rivara et al. 1989) and are available from several sources (see additional sources of information). World-class racers and other famous sports figures can be featured.

News stories about bicyclists who have suffered head injury can emphasize the worth of helmets. Since children ride bicycles most commonly in the warm months, attention from the media in late winter or early spring and continuing through the summer is well timed. Producers and photographers can help to change the public image of the all-American kid on a bike to include a helmet by picturing children riding helmeted. The acceptance of bicycle helmets by children and their parents will take time. A multifaceted educational approach in which members of the media play a crucial role will help.

References

American Academy of Pediatrics. 1987. *Injury Control for Children and Youth.* Elk Grove Village, Ill.: American Academy of Pediatrics.

Bergman, AB, et al. 1990. The Seattle children's Bicycle Helmet Campaign. *Am J Dis Child* 144:727-731.

Blomberg, RD, et al. 1986. Experimental evaluation of alternative conspicuity-enhancement techniques for pedestrians and bicyclists. *Journal of Safety Research* 17:1-12.

Burgess, B, and Burden, D. 1977. *Bicycle Safety and Information Report.* Prepared for the National Highway Traffic Safety Administration. Missoula, Mont.: Bikecentennial.

California. General Assembly. 1986. Assembly Bill No. 1019.

Consumer Product Safety Commission. 1988. Requirements for bicycles. 16 *CFR* 1500-1512.

Consumer Reports. 1990. Bike helmets: Unused lifesavers. *Consumer Reports* May: 348-353.

Dannenberg, AL. 1989. Bicycle safety helmets, letter. *N Engl J Med* 321(17):1195.

Dewar, RE. 1978. Bicycle riding practices: Implications for safety campaigns. *Journal of Safety Research* 11(1):35-42.

DiGuiseppi, CG, et al. 1989. Bicycle helmet use by children: Evaluation of a community-wide helmet campaign. *JAMA* 262(16):2256-2261.

Friede, AM, et al. 1985. The epidemiology of injuries to bicycle riders. *Pediatr Clin North Am* 32(1):141-152.

McFarlane, JP, et al. 1982. Injuries from bicycle accidents: The problem and recommended strategies for prevention. *Aust Paediatr J* 18(4):253-254.

National Center for Health Statistics. 1988. *Vital Statistics of the United States, 1986.* Vol. 2, Mortality, pt. A. Dept of Health and Human Services Publication No. (PHS) 88-1122. Washington, D.C.: U.S. Government Printing Office.

Rivara, FP, et al. 1989. Evaluation of potentially preventable deaths among pedestrian and bicyclist fatalities. *JAMA* 261(4):566-570.

Sandels, S. 1974. *Why Are Children Injured in Traffic: Can We Prevent Child Accidents in Traffic? The Skandia Report II.* Stockhkolm: Skandia Insurance Co. Ltd.

Selbst, SM, et al. 1987. Bicycle-related injuries. *Am J Dis Child* 141:140-144.

Sparnon, AL, and Ford, WD. 1986. Bicycle handlebar injuries in children. *J Pediatr Surg* 21(2):118-119.

Statewide Comprehensive Injury Prevention Program. 1983. Legislation – Bicycle safety. *SCIPP Reports* 4(2):9.

Thompson, RS, et al. 1989. A case-control study of the effectiveness of bicycle safety helmets. *N Engl J Med* 320(21):1361-1367.

Waller, JA. 1971. Bicycle ownership, use, and injury patterns among elementary school children. *Pediatrics* 47:1042-1050.

Washington Area Bicyclist Association. 1979. *Bicycle Helmet Wearability Study.* Washington, D.C.: Washington Area Bicyclist Association.

Watts, GR. 1983. *Pedal Cycle Spacers – A Study Involving School Children.* Transport and Road Research Laboratory Digest SR 801. Crowthorne, Berkshire, UK: Transport and Road Research Laboratory.

Weiss, BD, and Duncan, B. 1986. Bicycle helmet use by children: Knowledge and behavior of physicians. *Am J Public Health* 76(8):1022-1023.

Williams, J. 1984. Missoula Montana's bicycle helmet campaign: 1983-1984. *Bicycle Forum.*

Wood, T, and Milne, P. 1988. Head injuries to pedal cyclists and the promotion of helmet use in Victoria, Australia. *Accid Anal Prev* 20:177-185.

Additional Sources of Information

American Academy of Pediatrics (AAP)
141 Northwest Point Boulevard
PO Box 927
Elk Grove Village, IL 60009
312-228-5005
  Educational materials, including *Physician's Resource Guide for Bicycle Safety Education.*

American Association of State Highway and Transportation Officials (AASHTO)
444 North Capitol Street, NW, Suite 225
Washington, DC 20001
202-624-5800
  Materials on bicycle safety and facility design.

American Automobile Association (AAA)
Foundation for Traffic Safety
1730 M Street, NW
Suite 401
Washington, DC 20036
202-775-1456
  Educational materials and reports on bicycle safety and facility design.

American National Standards Institute (ANSI)
1430 Broadway
New York, NY 10018
212-354-3300
  Helmet standard (ANSI standard Z90.4-1984).

Bicycle Federation of America/
National Bicycle Education Consortium
1818 R Street, NW
Washington, DC 20009
202-332-6986
Educational materials.

Bicycle Helmet Safety Institute (a program of the Washington Area Bicyclist Association)
4611 Seventh Street South
Arlington, VA 22204
703-486-0100
Periodic updates on helmets, such as the Bicycle Helmet Workshop text with detailed information on helmets and testing, and various articles and materials, including a computerized documentation center.

Bikecentennial/Bicycle Forum
PO Box 8308
Missoula, MT 59807
406-721-1776
Educational materials, including bike rodeo guide.

Harborview Injury Prevention and Research Center
325 Ninth Avenue, ZX-10
Seattle, WA 98104
206-223-3158
PSAs, posters, and manuals describing community activities and school and PTA activities to promote helmet use.

League of American Wheelmen (LAW)
6707 Whitestone Road
Suite 209
Baltimore, MD 21207
301-944-3399
Materials on bicycle safety, including excerpt of Uniform Vehicle Code pertaining to bicycles.

Minnesota Community Bicycle Safety Program
University of Minnesota
4-H Youth Development
340 Coffey Hall
St. Paul, MN 55108
612-625-9719
Educational materials and manuals for community bike safety activities and bike patrols to enforce bicycle regulations.

National Highway Traffic Safety Administration (NHTSA)
400 7th Street, SW
Routing symbol NTS-23
Washington, DC 20590
202-366-2761
Educational materials and reports on bicycle safety and facility design.

National Safe Kids Campaign
Children's Hospital Medical Center
111 Michigan Avenue, NW
Washington, DC 20010
202-939-4993
Bike Helmet and Bike Safety Awareness Campaign guide, PSAs, posters, other educational materials.

Snell Memorial Foundation
PO Box 493
St. James, NY 11780
516-862-6545
Helmet standard.

Transportation Research Board (TRB)
National Research Council
2101 Constitution Avenue, NW
Washington, DC 20418
202-334-3214
Reports on bicycle safety and facility design.

III

THE HOME ENVIRONMENT

7

Fires and Burns

7.A Facts

House fires kill about 1,200 children aged 0–14 each year and account for 90% of all childhood burn deaths. House-fire death rates are especially high in the South and in low-income areas. In many states, more children die in house fires than as motor vehicle occupants or pedestrians. Most house-fire deaths result from the poisoning effects of smoke inhalation rather than from burn injury (Robinson and Seward 1987).

Death rates from house fires are similar for males and females except at ages 2–4, when the higher male death rates may reflect the greater tendency among boys to play with matches and cigarette lighters. The most common ignition source in house fires is a smoldering cigarette, typically leading to a slowly developing, nighttime fire in which carbon monoxide and other toxic fumes overcome children as they sleep. Other common ignition sources include flammable liquids (often used in arson) and kerosene or portable heaters.

Important measures for preventing house-fire deaths and injuries include installed, functioning smoke detectors and easy means of egress. Cigarettes can now be designed so they are less likely to ignite upholstered chairs and bedding (Technical Study Group 1987). Sprinkler systems for automatic fire extinguishment are increasingly cost-effective because they decrease property damage as well as saving lives; they are especially valuable because they will put out a fire. Unlike smoke detectors, their effectiveness does not depend on someone being present and able to respond to a crisis (Mulrine 1981).

Clothing ignition, once a prominent source of fatal burn injury, has been reduced by flame-retardant materials as mandated for children's sleepwear (McLoughlin et al. 1977). Also, tight-fitting clothing styles rather than loose or bouffant dresses and the use of synthetic fabrics that have less tendency to ignite upon contact with flame have reduced clothing-associated burns.

Children who survive house fires or clothing ignition are apt to have burns over large parts of their bodies. Extensive disfigurement and disability are likely to result, particularly when the face, hands, or genitals are involved. Severe burns may require dozens of operations, and their long-term costs and human consequences can devastate entire families.

Scalds are rarely a cause of death but are very important because of their high incidence in young children. Among children aged 0–4, more than 100,000 scalds each year require emergency room treatment, based on estimates from northeastern Ohio (Chatterjee et al. 1986). The highest incidence is at ages 1 and 2. Hot tap water, coffee, and tea are the most common agents, with boiling water or food the most damaging. Scalds occurring when children upset containers of hot liquid often affect the face and hands, areas that are cosmetically or functionally very important.

The importance of water temperature is instructive (Moritz and Henriques 1947). For example, for adult skin, water at 119°F may cause pain but does not cause a burn. Water at 130°F produces first- or second-degree burns in 29 seconds. Water at 140°F allows only 3 seconds in which to escape serious harm. Children's skin is thinner and burns faster and at lower temperatures than adult skin (Feldman 1983). Dangerous hot-water temperatures at the tap are readily achieved by current water heaters and even mandated by regulation in some jurisdictions. For both unintentional and intentional tap-water scalds, discussed later, serious effects are most readily prevented by limiting hot-water temperatures to 120–125°F.

Electrical mouth burns, often disfiguring, are especially apt to result when toddlers mouth the female end of a live extension cord (Crikelair and Dhaliwal 1976). Contact burns may be caused by unprotected home heating devices as well as a host of other appliances with hot surfaces, such as irons, curling irons, and stoves.

Fireworks are another source of childhood burns. Regulations have been effective in reducing injuries due to fireworks: in states that allow a wide variety of fireworks to be sold for personal use, the fireworks injury rate is seven times the rate in more restrictive states (Berger 1985).

Although the great majority of childhood burns are unintentional, about 10–15% are intentionally inflicted by adults (Hight et al. 1979). Burns are sometimes inflicted in disciplinary situations, including toilet training (Feldman 1980). Many burns resulting from abuse show characteristic patterns, such as hot tap-water scalds of the buttocks or perineum and cigarette burns on the back of the hand. Inflicted burns are likely to involve children who have been abused previously and suggest an escalating pattern of assault. Burns associated with parental neglect often involve chaotic homes, family violence, socially isolated mothers, unemployment, and geographical mobility (Ayoub and Pfeifer 1979).

7.B Developmental Considerations
7.B.1 Infants

Several factors contribute to high rates of fatal burns in infancy. Infants are more likely to die than older children with comparable burns (Georgiade and Moylan 1985). Their lack of independent mobility prevents infants from escaping on their own from smoke or flames. They are therefore especially likely to die in house fires, even when others get out. Infants are, of course, extremely vulnerable to inflicted burns, particularly scalding. Their limited mobility makes it all but impossible for them to escape from attempts to scald them by immersion in hot water, for example. Small size brings additional risk: babies and toddlers are small enough to fit in thermal and microwave ovens, which have been used to inflict injury.

During the middle of the first year, babies begin to reach for everything. Contact and scald burns become prominent as babies touch hot surfaces or spill hot liquids on themselves. Such burns are even more common when babies increase their access to hot materials by crawling, creeping, and finally walking and climbing.

7.B.2 Toddlers

Toddlers, with their ever-increasing mobility, are able to involve themselves with hot water, open fires, stoves, hot objects on tables, and the like. In their never-ending exploration of the world, they may mouth live cords and suffer electrical burns or tip their walkers over the hearth and fall into the fireplace. They will also drink liquids that are dangerously hot; recently it has been recognized that toddlers may develop enough tissue swelling after drinking hot liquids to close their airway (Kulick et al. 1988).

This is the peak age for recognized inflicted burns. Misguided parents may deliberately burn an errant toddler to teach the meaning of "hot," and frustrated parents may inflict hot-water burns as punishment for toilet-training infractions. Young toddlers are unable to escape from hot bathwater as quickly as an older child or young adult, and need to put their hands down to push to standing. The skin of babies and toddlers burns more deeply and quickly and at lower temperatures than the thicker skin of adults (Feldman 1983).

7.B.3 Preschoolers

As children busy themselves imitating adults in their daily chores, the pattern of burns follows. Appliances the child wishes to master but is too young to manage safely (curling irons, stoves, barbecues, irons, etc.) become offenders. Matches and lighters attract.

Styles appear to markedly affect the likelihood of clothing-ignition burns. Loose-fitting clothing such as nightgowns and skirts appears to put girls at special risk when they are near stoves or flames (McLoughlin et al. 1977). Match play, on the other hand, increases the burn risk in boys.

Children in this age range have some ability to escape inflicted burns, and their verbal capacity may make it easier for them to communicate distress effectively to adults who are assaulting them.

7.B.4 Elementary School Ages

In addition to burns from household objects used as intended but without adequate skill, elementary school-age children are the youngest age-group likely to obtain or to be allowed to handle many types of fireworks. Where fireworks are available, burn injuries in this age-group are difficult to avoid because of a child's curiosity and eagerness to do "grown-up" things. A somewhat fearful fascination with fire and loud sounds is deep-seated.

Match play by boys of elementary school age is responsible for some clothing-ignition burns and some house fires. The "curiosity fire setters" are males in this age-group who typically have not been problem children but who set one fire, get scared, and summon help. The "pathological fire setters," on the other hand, are repeat offenders and are deeply disturbed (McLoughlin and Crawford 1985).

7.B.5 Young Adolescents

Very severe burns may result when flammable liquids such as gasoline are misused to encourage a smoldering fire, to commit arson, or as a cleaning fluid in an enclosed space, where the fumes can be ignited by a small flame or spark. Older male children and adolescents are often involved (McLoughlin and Crawford 1985). In addition, young adolescent males may climb towers carrying power lines and thus are a high-risk group for rare but extremely serious high-voltage electrical injury (McLoughlin and Crawford 1985; McLoughlin et al. 1976). Electrocution and serious burns due to power lines are also threats to young adolescents working on farms.

School-age children and adolescents also are the most likely candidates for self-inflicted burns, usually in the context of psychiatric disorders. Finally, inflicted burns may occur even in older children and adolescents as assault (Feldman 1980) or as part of gang-related rituals.

Young adolescents who ride motorized cycles and similar vehicles may suffer leg burns from unprotected exhaust systems. In addition, the home responsibilities and first job opportunities for many may involve food preparation, which carries a high risk of burns.

7.C Opportunities for Protection

STRATEGIES FOR PREVENTING INJURIES FROM FIRES AND BURNS
(high-priority strategies are indicated by a △)

Changing Sources of Fires and Burns
- △ Mandate firesafe cigarettes.
- △ Develop childproof cigarette lighters.
- △ Ban use of fireworks except in community displays.

△ Ensure that water heaters or antiscald devices keep temperatures at the sink, tub, or shower below 125°F.
Use stable, shielded heaters and stoves.

Reducing Flammability
Use flame-retardant materials.
Design and choose close-fitting clothing.

Increasing Ability to Escape
△ Install smoke detectors that are wired into the electrical system.
Modify materials to reduce toxicants produced by burning.
Design housing to provide alternate escape routes.
Train children to plan for escape and to crawl under smoke.

Extinguishing Fires
△ Require automatic sprinkler systems in all dwellings.
Install fire extinguishers in kitchens, cars, and other high- risk areas.
Teach children to drop and roll if clothing catches fire.

Changing Adult Behavior
Discourage "teaching" children through contact with hot surfaces.
Develop fire-escape plans.
Maintain heating system, electrical appliances, low hot-water temperature.

Improving Emergency Care
△ Educate public to "cool a burn."
Provide adequate community fire-response system.
Teach personnel to recognize and report inflicted burn patterns.

7.C.1 Schools and Child Care Centers

Schools and child care centers need the same basic fire-prevention measures as other public buildings. In addition, schools need easy means of egress for any disabled and young students and an emergency fire plan that includes regular fire drills for all students and staff. Schools or child care centers with deaf students or teachers need fire alarms with flashing lights as well as auditory alarms. Prevention of fires, burns, and explosions should be a major consideration when planning or evaluating school science laboratories, home economics kitchens, industrial arts workshops, art classrooms, and stage productions.

Child care center personnel should routinely check for burn hazards, such as electrical cords dangling from coffee pots or teapots that could be pulled by a child, and should have a designated area where hot liquids such as coffee or tea will be out of the reach of small children. Food should be carefully cooled, and activities that might lead to fires or burns should be avoided.

Child care workers and teachers should take note of the presence of burns and burn scars on children, which may be a sign of maltreatment. A pattern of repeated injury is usually a danger signal. School personnel are obligated to inform the appropriate agency when maltreatment is suspected (see chapter 13).

Manuals outlining safe practices in school science laboratories are available and should be followed concerning lab facilities, equipment, and work habits (NIOSII 1980a; NIOSH 1980b; CSSS 1984). Science teachers and substitutes should be trained in safe laboratory procedures (including recognition of explosive or corrosive substances and safe storage, disposal, and substitution) and in first aid and cardiopulmonary resuscitation (CPR). Protective safety wear should be required for all persons working with hazardous substances (e.g., ANSI or equivalent standard-approved eye or face protection, no open-toed shoes). Particular attention should be given to the use of open flames (e.g., Bunsen burners) in science labs.

Severe burns have been reported among students who used dental plaster to make molds of their hands, in some cases resulting in finger amputation because of irreversible tissue damage. Plaster of paris can also cause severe burns (Hedeboe et al. 1982; Miller-Larsen et al. 1981).

Many curricula and teachers' guides for fire and burn prevention are in use, designed to affect students' attitudes, knowledge, and actions. For example, "Learn Not to Burn," a curriculum developed by the National Fire Protection Association for schoolchildren in kindergarten through eighth grade, features 25 key fire-safety skills to be integrated into regular school subject areas (CDC 1987). Some programs involve community figures, such as fire department and burn facility personnel, who present fire- and burn-prevention education to school, parent-teacher, and community groups (Mieszala and O'Connell 1982).

Educational burn-prevention programs should emphasize drop-and-roll techniques, cool-a-burn first aid techniques, planning fire-escape routes for school and home, and rules for escape from burning buildings, including crawling under smoke (McLoughlin and Crawford 1985). Educational efforts may increase knowledge among certain students, but a favorable effect on burn morbidity and mortality has not been clearly proven. One evaluation of school-based educational efforts showed no reduction in burn incidence and severity (MacKay and Rothman 1982; McLoughlin et al. 1982). Because there are many competing needs, additions to the curriculum aimed at reducing fires and burns deserve creative innovation, careful evaluation, and supplementation with other community programs. Education can be seen as only one part of a burn-prevention program.

Special efforts should be made to protect children in self-care (latchkey) arrangements. Some neglect-related burn cases involve inappropriate supervision of young children by school-age siblings. Though adult supervision is preferable, it is not always obtainable; training children to respond in the event of fires and burns is one way of helping both children in self-care and older children who are caring for younger siblings (Jones et al. 1981).

Since many serious fires are ignited by cigarettes, smoking by students and faculty alike should be severely restricted or prohibited.

7.C.2 Health Care Providers

Within their larger responsibility to be attentive to child maltreatment and its predisposing risk factors, health care providers must be acutely attentive to signs of inadequate or deteriorating care on the part of parents and be cognizant of the patterns associated with inflicted burns (Feldman 1980; Hight et al. 1979). Health care providers may also model good burn-prevention practices in their offices and, as a part of anticipatory guidance, may caution parents to be sure their hot-water temperature is no more than 125°F; to install and maintain smoke detectors; to cool burns as first aid; to plan and practice a fire-escape route from the home; and to teach children to crawl under smoke and to drop and roll if clothing is on fire.

Vaporizers recommended for young patients with colds should be the cool-mist type. Steam-mist vaporizers should be strongly discouraged; steam provides no additional efficacy but does carry the risk of burns from hot liquids.

Electrical burns and at least one electrocution have resulted from misconnections of home cardiopulmonary monitor electrode leads or power cords by a child (the patient or a sibling) (Katcher et al. 1986). Design changes could prevent similar events (see section 7.C.7). Parents should be advised to prevent access to wall outlets and to disconnect the lead wires from the child when the monitor is not in use. Only a trained adult should make the connections. The need for monitoring should be reassessed periodically with a view to its safety when the child becomes old enough to tamper with the equipment.

7.C.3 Public Agencies

To prevent fire and burn injury, agencies can establish housing or sanitary codes or strengthen and enforce existing codes. Aspects to be considered include easy and well-lighted egress, wiring, tap-water temperatures, and installation and maintenance of appliances and heating devices. Agencies should require day care centers, schools, foster homes, and other public buildings to install and maintain smoke detectors, sprinkler systems, fire escapes, and fire extinguishers, and to plan and post fire-escape routes. Inspections should be carried out routinely, with notification of violations sent to landlords and prompt reinspections. Regulatory measures combined with inspections and court hearings if necessary (even though costly and time-consuming) have been most effective in reducing hazards (Hunter 1983).

Agency personnel who make home visits should check equipment —

monitors, steam vaporizers, heating pads, and space heaters—that might cause burns or fires and can also check the hot-water temperature and help to turn down the water heater setting if necessary.

Agencies responsible for community planning, zoning, and transportation can work to be sure emergency fire equipment and personnel are appropriately placed. This requires reevaluation of existing conditions as populations change and may sometimes be accomplished by reallocating resources, without large expenditures.

High rates of house-fire deaths in rural areas may be due in part to delays in emergency equipment reaching the fire and delays in emergency medical care. In rural areas, grid mapping that allows easier location of the house fire should be established, year-round fire-road accessibility is necessary, and location of water supplies for pumping should be determined.

Fire departments have sponsored very successful programs to encourage householders to install smoke detectors, sometimes helping with installation or even giving them to residents free of charge (Gorman et al. 1985). Fire fighters can also be active in programs for arson prevention and fire setters. Fire departments can work with state and local agencies, police departments, prosecutors, insurance and banking representatives, municipal officials, and voluntary organizations to prevent arson. Aspects of intervention include early-warning systems, arson-prevention and arson-detection programs, successful prosecution, and efforts focused on identifying juvenile fire setters and responding to their needs.

Protective-service agencies must be prepared to deal with inflicted burns as an expression of child maltreatment. Studies indicate that families who inflict burns on their children often have had prior protective-services contact (Ayoub and Pfeifer 1979). Thus, burns in these cases reflect a failure to intervene adequately with these children and families. Additional strategies must be devised and evaluated.

Protective-service personnel can help others who deal with children to recognize inflicted burns, such as scalds of the genitals and cigarette burns (Hight et al. 1979; Feldman 1980). Agencies can push for standards for adult supervision, suggesting an age below which children are not to be left unsupervised.

7.C.4 Legislators and Regulators

Legislators can work for building and housing codes that address fire and burn prevention. Sprinkler systems are required by some jurisdictions in new multifamily dwellings and should be required in all new dwellings; retrofitting might be considered in rental units of any age. Subsidies are likely to be helpful. Smoke detectors should be required in all new and existing dwellings. Consistent regulation is needed concerning fire escapes, codes for wiring, water heater temperatures, and fire extinguishers. Home heating standards are needed, along with comprehensive regulations governing kerosene and wood-burning stoves. Legislation needs to address adequate enforcement as well. For example, compliance was difficult to obtain with a Massachusetts law requiring smoke detectors that relied on local fire departments for enforcement, since they in turn relied on private interest groups such as banking and real estate personnel. Shifting the responsibility for enforcement to local boards of health may be a successful alternative (Miclette 1982).

Legislation supported by some members of the U.S. Congress and legislators in several states would require that only firesafe cigarettes (those with a lowered propensity to ignite house fires) be manufactured and sold in the United States (Technical Study Group 1987).

The CPSC should consider expanding its standard for flame-retardant sleepwear for children to include other garments. Currently, garments used for sleepwear but labeled by the manufacturers as long underwear do not comply.

The Consumer Product Safety Commission should require disposable butane lighters to be child-resistant. In a 1987 CPSC study, disposable butane lighters were found to be a primary source of cigarette-lighter fires (CPSC 1987). Children who operated the lighters were usually less than 6 years old, primarily 3- and 4-year-olds; their parents either did not realize their children could operate the lighters or did not appreciate the danger.

State legislation restricting the sale of fireworks has proved effective in preventing burns and fires (Berger et al. 1985). A wide range of fireworks sales to individuals are permitted in some states; easy access to fireworks in neighboring states may reduce the efficacy of laws in those states that do restrict sales. As of 1988, two states did not have any state fireworks regulations at all. Twenty-eight states allowed private use of some or all types of "Class C" fireworks—those classified as "common fireworks" by the U.S. Department of Transportation in the Code of Federal Regulations, including cone fountains, Roman candles, sky rockets, firecrackers, and certain sparklers. Only 13 states banned all Class C fireworks (National Council on Fireworks Safety 1988). Federal legislation prohibiting the sale of all Class C fireworks to private individuals would be helpful in further reducing the number of fireworks-related injuries and fires.

Legislation mandating minimum ages at which children can be left without adult supervision might help to prevent neglect-related burns and house-fire deaths of unattended children.

7.C.5 Law Enforcement Professionals

Law enforcement officers often are called to respond to situations of domestic violence, which may be a feature common to neglect-related burn cases. In addition to being trained as first responders to provide emergency medical assistance, officers should be trained to examine any children they encounter in responding to domestic violence calls for evidence of abuse, including old or healing burns. Early recognition can be lifesaving since, in the case of children hospitalized for abuse- or neglect-related burns, the burn for which a child is hospitalized is rarely the first burn and almost never the first significant injury sustained by the child at home (Feldman 1980; Hight et al. 1979).

Law enforcement officers may be involved in enforcing regulations pertaining to fire and burn prevention, such as confiscating illegal fireworks and apprehending child arsonists. Training and educational programs can be conducted to make personnel aware of the devastating effects of fires and burns, developmental considerations concerning children that may make them likely to start a fire or unable to escape, and the importance of fire and burn prevention.

7.C.6 Voluntary Organizations

Organizations can push to limit the sales of fireworks to individuals and can provide supervised displays for groups under carefully controlled conditions. Smoke detectors given away by a fire department have been installed and maintained by residents of high-risk housing (Gorman et al. 1985); there are no obvious reasons why voluntary organizations could not succeed with a similar program. Providing easily installed smoke detectors at a small cost, rather than for free, may actually result in a higher rate of use. People at both ends of the age spectrum, the elderly as well as young children, are particularly likely to die in a house fire or to suffer burn injury. Community initiatives aimed at protecting senior citizens with smoke detectors or lowered water heater temperatures, for instance, are likely to benefit children as well.

Groups who provide programs for children can include curricular units on fire and burn prevention and first aid. Community-based support groups for abusive parents have been organized in some areas (see chapter 13). Their success in reducing burn injuries is unknown.

7.C.7 Designers, Architects, Builders, and Engineers

Automatic sprinkler systems, smoke detectors which are connected into the electrical system, and easy egress should be part of all new building plans. Inexpensive antiscald devices can be installed in hot-water taps to prevent discharge of water that exceeds a specified temperature. Ground fault circuit interrupters (GFCIs) — inexpensive, easily installed electrical devices which switch off power to a circuit when current loss is detected — can prevent electrocutions and electric shocks (CPSC 1985). GFCIs are required by some building codes; their use in bathrooms, kitchens, garages, basements, and outdoor outlets should be standard practice. Housing incorporating new technologies, such as the "Smart House" project of the National Association of Home Builders' National Research Center, may help reduce injuries due to house fires and burns in the future.

Enthusiasm for developing flame-retardant fabrics was affected in the 1970s by the finding that tris(hydroxymethyl)amino methane (TRIS) may have carcinogenic potential (Bergman 1977; Crikelair 1980). This should not prevent development of new retardants and increasingly protective standards for clothing, drapery, mattresses, upholstery, and building materials. Often the characteristics of the fabric—tightness of weave, nap, etc.—can be altered to diminish flammability without requiring the addition of chemicals. In addition, since most persons appear to succumb to toxic gas inhalation before flames reach them, the toxicants produced by burning materials might be deliberately reduced. In addition to fabric characteristics, the design of children's clothes affects the potential for ignition. Close-fitting styles of flame-retardant materials are safest. Labeling that reflects gradations in flammability has been suggested (CDC 1978).

Plastic caps or a nonconductive cuff attached to the female end of extension cords could prevent electrical mouth burns to toddlers (Crikelair and Dhaliwal 1976). Electrical appliances should be designed with cords that cannot dangle within the reach of a young child. Options include cords that are short or coiled, or cords that retract automatically.

Home cardiopulmonary monitors intended for use with infants and small children should be designed so that inappropriate connections resulting in the flow of electricity to the child are not possible. Design changes include making the power cord a permanent part of the monitor so that the electrode leads cannot be plugged directly into the power cord and designing the leads so they cannot be inserted into the power cord, an extension cord, or a wall socket (Katcher et al. 1986).

Kitchen layouts that are attentive to "traffic" patterns can reduce the likelihood that pans of hot liquids or foods will be lifted over the heads of young children. Easy-to-install barriers are needed to keep toddlers away from hot surfaces (floor furnace grates, wood stoves, radiators, etc.). Since children are often burned when families cook outdoors, barbecue facilities and appliances should be designed to prevent child contact with fuel or hot surfaces.

Children are often rear-seat occupants of passenger cars and thus are particularly vulnerable when a rear-end collision ignites gasoline from the gas tank of the leading car. Gas-tank design changes might make such ignition less likely. Exhaust systems for vehicles such as mopeds and motorbikes should be guarded to prevent leg burns.

7.C.8 Business and Industry

The two measures most likely to reduce childhood mortality from house fires and burns are automatic sprinkler systems and the replacement of current cigarettes with firesafe cigarettes. Lowering insurance premiums for sprinkler-protected buildings might stimulate the proliferation of this cost-saving investment. Firesafe cigarettes are much less likely to ignite materials than current cigarettes and would avert much human and property damage.

The voluntary agreement of the Gas Appliances Manufacturers' Association (GAMA) to preset the temperature of water heaters at a relatively safe 125°F and provide warning labels and installation instructions is a positive first step in reducing scald injuries. The next step is to manufacture water heaters that can supply adequate volumes of hot water that never exceeds 125°F at the tap.

High-voltage power-line towers and other sources of electricity should be made inaccessible to exploring youths.

7.C.9 Mass Media

A number of simple messages which might prevent fire deaths and burn injuries are appropriate to present to the public in the mass media. Among them would be the importance of installing and maintaining smoke detectors and responding to their alarm; to leave the scene of a fire and summon help rather than try to fight an uncontrollable fire, even with a fire extinguisher; to "stop, drop, and roll" when clothing ignites; to avoid playing with fireworks; to cool a burn as first aid; safe use of outdoor grills; home heating issues; and the effectiveness and economy of sprinkler systems and safe water heater settings. Obviously, some of these are appropriate for repetition on a seasonal basis.

A second important area of emphasis for the mass media is to convey the importance of adult supervision for all children as a minimum standard of care. Such supervision is needed for many reasons, but especially pertinent here is the likelihood of averting some deaths from house fires which occur while unattended children sleep and fires and burns which occur when unsupervised children play with matches or other hot objects.

House fires are very frequently "news" in urban areas. When house-fire stories are featured, prevention can be featured, too. Emphasizing the prime role of "cigarette-ignited fires" may prepare the public to accept or demand firesafe cigarettes. There has been little apparent preventive impact from labeling fires as "due to careless smoking"; the term should be replaced by "ignited by a smoldering cigarette."

Images of people smoking that might be construed as positive and therefore might encourage smoking should be avoided when possible. Smoking has many negative effects on health, but most important here is the fact that cigarettes cause many fires which result in personal injury.

References

Ayoub, C, and Pfeifer, D. 1979. Burns as a manifestation of child abuse and neglect. *Am J Dis Child* 133:910–914.

Berger, LR, et al. 1985. Injuries from fireworks. *Pediatrics* 75(5):877–882.

Bergman, AG. 1977. Flame-resistant sleepwear: Have the bird-watchers gone ape? *Pediatrics* 60(4 pt.2):652–654.

Centers for Disease Control. 1987. *Prevention of Injuries to Children and Youth:*

A Selected Bibliography. Atlanta: U.S. Dept. of Health and Human Services.
Centers for Disease Control. 1978. *An Epidemiologic Study of Burn Injuries and Strategies for Prevention.* Report prepared by Feck et al. Atlanta: Centers for Disease Control.
Chatterjee, BF, et al. 1986. Northeastern Ohio Trauma Study: V. Burn injury. *J Trauma* 26(9):844.
Consumer Product Safety Commission. 1985. *Ground Fault Circuit Interrupters (GFCI).* Product Safety Fact Sheet No. 99. Washington, D.C.: Consumer Product Safety Commission.
Consumer Product Safety Commission. 1987. *Fire Hazards Involving Children Playing with Cigarette Lighters.* Report prepared by B. Harwood. Washington, D.C.: Consumer Product Safety Commission.
Council of State Science Supervisors. 1984. *School Science Laboratories: A Guide to Some Hazardous Substances.* Washington, D.C.: Consumer Product Safety Commission.
Crikelair, GF. 1980. Anti-Trisers—Where are you?, letter. *Pediatrics* 66(6):1027-1028.
Crikelair, GF, and Dhaliwal, AS. 1976. The cause and prevention of electrical burns of the mouth in children: A protective cuff. *Plast Reconstr Surg* 58(2):206-209.
Feldman, KW. 1983. Help needed on hot water burns, letter. *Pediatrics* 71(1):145-146.
Feldman, KW. 1980. Child abuse by burning, in Kempe, CH, and Helfer, RE (eds.): *The Battered Child*, ed. 3. Chicago: University of Chicago Press, pp. 147-162.
Georgiade, GS, and Moylan, J. 1985. Burns, in Mayer, TA (ed.): *Emergency Management of Pediatric Trauma.* Philadelphia: WB Saunders Co., pp. 413-420.
Gorman, RL, et al. 1985. A successful city-wide smoke detector giveaway program. *Pediatrics* 75(1):14-18.
Hedeboe J, et al. 1982. Heat generation in plaster-of-Paris and resulting hand burns. *Burns Incl Therm Inj* 9(1):46-48.
Hight, DW, et al. 1979. Inflicted burns in children: Recognition and treatment. *JAMA* 242:517-520.
Hunter, P. 1983. Reducing hazards in the home. *SCIPP Reports* 4(1):10.
Jones, RT, et al. 1981. Social validation and training of emergency fire safety skills for potential injury prevention and life saving. *J Appl Behav Anal* 14(3):249-260.
Katcher, ML, et al. 1986. Severe injury and death associated with home infant cardiorespiratory monitors. *Pediatrics* 78(5):775-779.
Kulick, RM, et al. 1988. Thermal epiglottitis after swallowing hot beverages. *Pediatrics* 81(3):441-444.
MacKay, AM, and Rothman, KJ. 1982. The incidence and severity of burn injuries following Project Burn Prevention. *Am J Public Health* 72(3):248-252.
McLoughlin, E, and Crawford, JD. 1985. Burns. *Pediatr Clin North Am* 32(1):61-76.
McLoughlin, E, et al. 1982. Project Burn Prevention: Outcome and implications. *Am J Public Health* 72(3):241-247.
McLoughlin, E, et al. 1977. One pediatric burn unit's experience with sleepwear-related injuries. *Pediatrics* 60(4):405-409.

McLoughlin, E, et al. 1976. Epidemiology of high-tension electrical injuries in children. *J Pediatr* 89(1):62-65.

Miclette, M. 1982. Legislation. *SCIPP Reports* 3(1):9.

Mieszala, P, and O'Connell, TJ. 1982. Burn center-fire department joint effort in fire prevention education. *J Burn Care Rehabil* 3(5):294.

Miller-Larsen, F, et al. 1981. [Hand burns caused by dental plaster]. *Ugeskr Laeger* 143(50):3386-3388.

Moritz, AR, and Henriques, FC. 1947. Studies of thermal injury: II. The relative importance of time and surface temperature in the causation of cutaneous burns. *Am J Pathol* 23:695-720.

Mulrine, JF. 1981. *Fire Sprinkler Laws: A Legislative Guide to Their Development.* Patterson, N.Y.: National Automatic Sprinkler and Fire Control Association, Inc.

National Council on Fireworks Safety. 1988. *Fireworks in America: Safety Information.* Washington, D.C.: American Pyrotechnics Association.

National Institute for Occupational Safety and Health. 1980a. *Manual of Safety and Health Hazards in the School Science Laboratory.* Washington, D.C.: U.S. Dept. of Health and Human Services.

National Institute for Occupational Safety and Health. 1980b. *Safety in the School Science Laboratory.* Cincinnati.

Robinson, MD, and Seward, PN. 1987. Hazardous chemical exposure in children. *Pediatr Emerg Care* 3(3):179-183.

Technical Study Group on Cigarette and Little Cigar Fire Safety. 1987. *Toward a less fire-prone cigarette.* Final report. Washington, D.C.: Consumer Product Safety Commission.

Additional Sources of Information

American Academy of Pediatrics (AAP)
141 Northwest Point Boulevard
PO Box 927
Elk Grove Village, IL 60009
312-228-5005
State legislative packet on regulating residential water heaters includes model legislation.

Center for Fire Research
National Institute of Standards and Technology
Fire Research Information Services
Building 224, Room A-252
Gaithersburg, MD 20899
301-975-6860
Technical reports and FIREDOC, a computerized bibliographic search service.

International Association of Chiefs of Police
1110 North Glebe Road
Suite 200
Arlington, VA 22201
Information for law enforcement professionals on arson.

National Association of Home Builders' National Research Center
400 Prince George's Boulevard
Upper Marlboro, MD 20772
301-249-4000
Information on advanced housing technologies.

National Committee for Prevention of Child Abuse
332 South Michigan Avenue
Suite 1250
Chicago, IL 60604
312-663-3520
"When School's Out and Nobody's Home," booklet on latchkey arrangements.

National Criminal Justice Reference Service
National Institute of Justice
Box 6000
Rockville, MD 20850
800-851-3420 or 301-251-5500 (in Maryland)
Information on arson.

National Fire Protection Association (NFPA)
1 Batterymarch Park
Quincy, MA 02269
617-770-3000
Educational materials, including *Learn Not to Burn* curriculum, and information for design and construction of buildings, including *Life Safety Code* (NFPA 101).

National Fire Sprinkler Association, Inc.
PO Box 1000
Patterson, NY 12563
914-878-4200
Information on fire sprinkler systems, including building codes and legislation.

National Smoke, Fire and Burn Institute
90 Sargent Road
Brookline, MA 02146
617-426-3161
Educational materials and films.

Network for Injury Prevention in Buildings (NIP)
Box 67, Blue Ridge Hospital
University of Virginia Medical Center
Charlottesville, VA 22901
804-924-5308
Information on model building codes.

8

Poisoning

8.A Facts

One of the most encouraging trends in childhood mortality is the reduction in deaths from poisoning. In 1960 there were 445 poisoning deaths in children younger than 5 years; in 1986 there were only 59. Although poisoning is no longer a major cause of death in very young children, it remains an important cause of hospitalizations and medical visits. Data from the state of Maryland, for instance, suggest that for every poisoning death in the under-5 age-group about 250 poisoned children are admitted to hospitals (Trinkoff and Baker 1986).

The substances most commonly ingested by the Maryland children were aspirin, solvents and petroleum products, tranquilizers, and iron compounds, with the highest rates seen in children about 1–2 years old; boys were at slightly higher risk than girls. Among teenagers, aspirin and psychoactive drugs (tranquilizers, sedatives, and antidepressants) were most commonly used. Females had the highest rates, and half of the poisonings were suicide attempts. An additional one-fourth were of unknown intent. Other studies have found similar patterns in hospitalized youngsters.

The extent of the poisoning problem cannot be appreciated fully from the number of deaths and hospital admissions. Some 700,000 cases of poisoning in the under-5 age-group were reported in 1987 by the poison-control centers participating in the American Association of Poison Control Centers (AAPCC) National Data Collection System. These centers serve just under 60% of the U.S. population. About 90,000 cases were reported for ages 5–12 and 50,000 for ages 13–17 (Litovitz et al. 1988).

Calls to poison-control centers following ingestions by children under 5 years of age reflect the availability of hazardous substances in children's environments. Many such calls are about fever or cough and cold preparations or other medicines, plants, cosmetics, or cleaning and polishing agents.

The reductions in poisoning deaths in young children are due to several factors, probably including poison-control centers and better emergency care, child-resistant packaging, reformulation of some poisonous substances such as lead paint, and reduced use of other substances such as kerosene.

Syrup of ipecac, an inexpensive, safe agent used to induce vomiting (and thereby to evacuate remaining poison with the stomach contents) is available without a prescription and should be kept for emergency use in homes with small children. Because vomiting could be dangerous in a few poisoning situations, ipecac should be administered at home only following telephone advice from a poison-control center or health care provider.

The proportions of child poisonings related to child abuse or neglect are not known. The failure of adults to meet minimal standards of substance storage and child supervision certainly plays a significant role in the overall problem. Outright assaults by poisoning are few in number but dramatic in their consequences. Thus, vigilance is warranted on the part of all those responsible for responding to poisonings. One danger sign is the repeater—the child who is seen more than once for ingestions. Whether it be poisonings, burns, or any other injury, a pattern of harm in a family should lead to a careful and sensitive investigation of family conditions, based on the assumption that multiple "accidents" may indicate the presence of neglect or even abuse. Ingestions among older children and adolescents may reflect serious depression on the child's part, and/or may be the outgrowth of living in an emotionally, sexually, or physically abusive family (Garbarino et al. 1986).

8.B Developmental Considerations

8.B.1 Infants

Very young infants, dependent on older persons for what goes into their mouths, are poisoned by adults, mostly unintentionally, through misuse or overuse of medications. Infants are particularly vulnerable to abusive poisonings because they cannot communicate directly about their experience. By 9 months of age, the child's routine mouthing of objects becomes the major source of risk. Independent mobility provided by crawling and then walking allows them to swallow drugs, household products, parts of plants, cosmetics, cigarettes, and the like. Careless storage of toxic substances becomes a salient issue as the child's capacity to reach and ingest substances increases.

8.B.2 Toddlers

Toddlers are at the highest risk for unintentional and repetitive poisoning. At this age the child's mobility increases, and curiosity definitely exceeds ability to assess risks. Toddlers are too young to benefit from poison-prevention labeling and education themselves. They depend on adult supervision and the safety of their environment for protection, and this makes them acutely vulnerable to neglectful injury.

8.B.3 Preschoolers

During the preschool period, children remain quite vulnerable to poisoning dangers because of their continuing exploratory behavior and play. They love to mimic adult behavior and may even ingest dangerous substances while playing "house." Children in families with drug- and alcohol-abusing adults may be at special risk.

8.B.4 Elementary School Ages

By elementary school age most children are capable of discriminating between dangerous and benign ingestible substances. Thus, the risk of accidental poisoning of the type common in early childhood declines.

8.B.5 Young Adolescents

By early adolescence the risk of intentional self-poisoning, including carbon monoxide poisoning from auto exhaust, use of drugs and alcohol, and workplace exposures, becomes evident as children take on increasingly adultlike attitudes and behaviors.

8.C Opportunities for Protection

> STRATEGIES FOR PREVENTING POISONINGS
> (high-priority strategies indicated by a △)
>
> *Decreasing the Supply of Poison*
>
> △ Limit the total dose in a single medication container.
> Limit the number of drugs available without prescription.
> Prescribe fewer medications, smaller doses, shorter time courses, and fewer refills.
> Develop and use alternatives to toxic household products such as kerosene.
>
> *Restricting Access to Poison*
>
> △ Install an easily accessible, easily locked and unlocked cabinet in all homes.
> Keep toxic materials in original containers, labeled with clear warnings, closed with child-resistant caps, and stored out of the reach of children.
> Change packaging to make medications and other toxic materials less attractive and more difficult to reach (individual-dose packaging, amber bottles, child-resistant caps, etc.).
> Expand the number of products required by the Poisoning Prevention Packaging Act to have child-resistant closures.
> Ensure that children have their medications administered by an adult.
> Make sure that exhaust systems for vehicles and heating units vent toxic inhalants (like carbon monoxide) away from occupants.

Reducing the Motivation for Poisoning
> Improve recognition of and treatment for suicidal adolescents and abusing caregivers.
>
> Make poisonous substances taste bad or appear less attractive.

Clearing Poison from the Body before It Is absorbed
> Make syrup of ipecac more widely available and standardize labeling.
>
> Administer syrup of ipecac when indicated.
>
> Improve the palatability of activated charcoal.
>
> Improve access to and performance of poison-control centers.

8.C.1 Schools and Child Care Centers

Elementary schoolchildren are not in a high-risk group for either unintentional or suicidal poisoning. While poison-prevention educational units have been designed for elementary schoolchildren and, if effective, might benefit younger siblings, the programs are unlikely to have a direct effect on the most urgent aspects of the poisoning problem, and should not displace injury-control topics of more urgency for the age-group being educated.

Elementary schoolchildren should not be directly responsible for the care of younger children or the administration, storage, or use of medications or other hazardous substances. Medications taken at school should be administered under the supervision of a school nurse or other specified adult. Diabetics, asthmatics, and other children taught to administer their own medications should still be supervised by an adult.

Early adolescent poisonings represent, almost exclusively, suicidal gestures or attempts. Schoolteachers should be made aware of the signs of depression during adolescence and should take threats of suicide seriously. Easy access to evaluation and counseling should be assured. Suicide-prevention guidelines for schools are discussed further in section 14.C.1.

Although unintentional poisoning at school or with school materials is not common, it may occur in school science laboratories. Hazardous-substance guidelines are available from the Council of State Science Supervisors (CSSS 1984) and may have an impact on burn injuries as well as on poisonings. School bus exhaust systems should be designed and maintained to minimize carbon monoxide exposure to passengers.

Nursery school and day care settings for young children are a different matter in regard to poisoning. Toddlers are at highest risk for unintentional poisoning, and all hazardous materials must be clearly marked, kept in their original containers (so they do not find their way into food and drink by mistake), and stored out of reach. Day care regulations should specify safe storage, and sites should be inspected frequently for violations. The training of day care personnel and of parents licensed to care for other children in their homes should include safe storage of hazardous materials and first aid procedures for poisoning. Phone access to a regional poison-control center should be assured, and syrup of ipecac should be available on-site. Adults should be instructed to call a poison-control center *before* administering syrup of ipecac, since making the child vomit is sometimes unnecessary and occasionally dangerous, such as after ingestion of caustic substances.

8.C.2 Health Care Providers

Historically, pediatricians, pharmacists, and federal health agencies have been leaders in the movement to prevent childhood poisoning. Opportunities continue to exist. Since most serious poisonings in childhood are related to unintended ingestion by the child of a medication used by someone else in the household, the most effective methods of prevention are likely to be those that most effectively decrease the availability of medications, that is, decreasing the number of medications prescribed and the quantities prescribed to the safest minimum and then providing them in child-resistant containers. (It is probably foolhardy to consider any container "child-proof.") Physicians and pharmacists should be informed about and comply with the regulations of the Poison Prevention Packaging Act (CPSC 1986), should encourage patients to accept child-resistant packaging, and should recommend strict storage practices to patients who request noncomplying containers because they have difficulty opening child-resistant containers. Health care providers have a direct impact on the quantity of medications in the environment because they prescribe them. The potential for unintentional ingestion should be kept in mind and prescribing limited. Many medications and other preparations for use with animals are toxic to children. Veterinarians should dispense products in child-resistant containers and warn animal owners (Glickman et al. 1982).

Health care providers play an important role in preventing absorption of poison after it has been ingested. Though long debated, syrup of ipecac appears to be a safe and effective way to rid the stomach of most poisons when ingestion is detected soon after it takes place. Most children come to medical attention within 2 hours of ingestion. The severity of the poisoning can be decreased by the rapid administration of ipecac. The earliest administration can take place at home, making the availability of ipecac in the home desirable. The office of the health care provider is an important place to distribute ipecac (or to encourage its purchase), since the peak age for unintentional ingestions is between 1 and 2 years. At that age most children are still making regular visits to the health care provider, who can distribute or recommend ipecac and educate the parent to call a poison-control center or an emergency service before using it since vomiting is sometimes contraindicated.

Deliberate poisoning of a child by a caregiver should be suspected when a symptom complex is poorly explained (e.g., unexplained episodes of loss of consciousness or seizures) or when symptoms disappear after admission or recur only when the parent is with the child. Although a wide range of substances has been associated with abusive poisoning, forced salt or water ingestion have been most commonly recognized. Repeated episodes of poisoning leading to clinical symptoms are a common form of "Munchausen Syndrome by Proxy" (illness in a child that's been induced or fabricated by a parent), and the index of suspicion must be high. Diagnosis and intervention can prevent future poisoning and abuse.

Early adolescents, like their older peers, may use intentional ingestion to threaten or accomplish suicide. Health care providers must develop and use methods to screen for, detect, and intervene with suicidal intent (see section 14.C.2). Early adolescents with chronic diseases requiring medication have a poison readily available. Instances of drug toxicity and overdose should be explored with a view to preventing future episodes. Prevention should not be forgotten when immediate medical needs have been addressed.

8.C.3 Public Agencies

Poison-control centers must meet the standards for regional centers established by the American Association of Poison Control Centers. Regional centers, which usually serve a population base of at least 1 million (McIntire and Angle 1983), have been shown to be more proficient than nonregional centers (Thompson et al. 1983).

Children from families experiencing a large number of disrupting life events (homelessness, unemployment, illness, or death, etc.) are particularly likely to be involved in ingestions. Agencies designing services for such families should include poison prevention in their programming. Parenting classes can also include poison prevention. Furthermore, foster homes and shelters should have arrangements so that poison hazards are eliminated (e.g., convenient locking cupboards or high shelves).

8.C.4 Legislators and Regulators

Federal attempts to prevent poisonings in the home began many years ago. The Caustic Poisons Act of 1927 required cautionary labeling of some corrosive substances and was later amended to ban household use of some particularly hazardous substances. Since World War II, requirements for labeling of toxic substances have been steadily broadened and strengthened under what is now known as the Federal Hazardous Substances Act. Nevertheless, as data from poison-control centers showed, childhood poisonings continued. Labeling was not enough to protect children. Hence, the Poison Prevention Packaging Act (PPPA), now administered by the CPSC, was passed in 1970 requiring that some toxic substances accessible to children be sold in containers difficult for a young child to open. Substances included under the PPPA as of 1988 were aspirin, some furniture polishes, methyl salicylate, controlled drugs, sodium and potassium hydroxide, kindling and illuminating preparations, methanol, sulfuric acid, most prescription drugs (although the consumer can request noncomplying packaging), ethylene glycol, iron-containing drugs and dietary supplements, solvents for paints and other "surface coatings," acetaminophen, and diphenhydramine hydrochloride (CPSC 1988). Packaging standards for pesticides are in the purview of the Environmental Protection Agency under the Federal Insecticide, Fungicide, and Rodenticide Act (FIFRA).

The PPPA should be updated periodically to include substances which continue to be a problem or newly marketed substances which come to be recognized as associated with hazardous ingestions and are not currently covered by the act. Some veterinary products (Glickman et al. 1982) and farm chemicals, such as dairy pipeline cleaners (Edmonson 1987), are examples.

Minimizing ingestion hazard should be a high priority when the regulation of drug sales is considered. Particularly hazardous medications should not be available without prescription. Over-the-counter medications should be packaged in amounts constituting a nonfatal total dose, should not be made attractive to children, and child-resistant packaging should be required (see section 8.C.7). Compliance by pharmacies with the specifications for the dispensing of medications is crucial (see CPSC 1986).

Kerosene in household use represents a severe poisoning hazard. Such use should be discouraged by regulation. New environmental regulations requiring conversion of vehicles from gas-powered to alternative fuel–powered engines may result in an increase in serious fuel poisonings, particularly among young adolescents. For example, methanol poisoning is more serious than gasoline poisoning (Litovitz 1988). Such trends should be studied after legislation is in place.

8.C.5 Law Enforcement Professionals

Panicked parents may call the police or fire department first in the event of a childhood poisoning. Personnel can be taught to contact the regional poison-control center to help guide their response. Additionally, personnel may be trained to identify, collect, and preserve any containers or soiled articles associated with the poisoning. These items are useful in identifying the substance and calculating the probable dose, and therefore in treating the child. They also may be useful in any subsequent investigation.

8.C.6 Voluntary Organizations

Community-based campaigns to raise awareness of poisoning as a hazard or, better yet, to eliminate specific poisoning hazards are probably more effective than broader, less targeted campaigns. Voluntary organizations can offer home-safety inspections to families with young children to help identify poisoning hazards as well as other home injury risks. Syrup of ipecac could be distributed free of charge. Organizations for farm families have a unique opportunity to educate members about the safe storage of agricultural liquids such as dairy pipeline cleaners (Edmonson 1987) and the hazards of manure pit and silo gases (Farm Safety Association 1985a, 1985b). Innovative community-based programs to prevent suicide are needed. Citizens of each community should demand toll-free phone access to a poison-control center which meets the standards for regional centers established by the American Association of Poison Control Centers.

8.C.7 Designers, Architects, Builders, and Engineers

Although closures cannot be expected to be absolutely "childproof," they should come very close. New designs for child-resistant caps for medication bottles and other hazardous substances would be welcomed. Current designs are often opened by children and are troublesome for adults. Child-resistant closures should stymie almost all young children but be relatively easy for most adults to open, even older adults with arthritis and diminished eyesight. If adults cannot easily work the devices, they leave them off or exercise their option to receive their prescription without a child-resistant cap, thus increasing the hazard for young visitors to their environment. Poisoning warning labels should be designed to be meaningful to people who cannot read English and to the visually impaired.

Unit-dose packaging of medications in plastic or foil serves as a barrier between the child and each dose of a medication, and would very likely decrease the total dose ingested. Amber or opaque bottling or foil unit packaging obscures the attractiveness of medications for children. Medications, including over-the-counter preparations and vitamins containing iron, should not be made to resemble candy.

Hazardous substances should be packaged in such a way that the consumer will not wish to or will be discouraged from transferring them to another container. Alternate containers are less likely to be clearly labeled and to have child-resistant closings and therefore promote unintentional poisonings.

Powders made for baby care present an inhalation hazard for the infant. Containers should be designed to permit the escape of no more than a small amount at a time.

Small, button-shaped batteries are easily swallowed by young children and contain corrosive chemicals which can cause perforation of the gastrointestinal tract. Such batteries should not be used in products designed for children. They should be protected from casual removal in products designed for adults.

Very alkaline substances (toilet bowl cleaners, for instance) cause substantial chemical burns to the mouth and esophagus when ingested, even in small amounts. When they are present in commonly used household substances, they are available to young children. Alternative products should be developed which do the job with less risk from ingestion. Some cosmetic products are highly toxic, such as false nail adhesive remover (Caravati and Litovitz 1988). Such products should be packaged with child-resistant closures and have graphic warning labels.

Cabinets intended for medication storage (bathroom "medicine" cabinets) or often used for poisonous household substances (under-the-sink cabinets) might have built-in child-resistant latching devices.

8.C.8 Business and Industry

Manufacturers' quality-control programs should be designed to eliminate the possibility of labeling errors, and the visibility, clarity, and effectiveness of warning labels can be improved.

Toxic fluids and their containers should not resemble edible fluids or their containers. The taste of hazardous fluids might be made obnoxious by the addition of substances which are not in themselves poisonous.

Materials made for the purpose of clearing the body of poison following ingestion (thereby decreasing the amount of poison absorbed) can be improved. Specifically, labeling of syrup of ipecac should be standardized, and activated charcoal could be made more palatable to children.

Manufacturers are responsible for supplying child-resistant packaging for prescription drugs and other substances covered by the PPPA that are dispensed to consumers. Manufacturers of hazardous household products not currently included under the PPPA and of toxic products not specifically designed for household use but likely to end up being available to children should voluntarily supply child-resistant packaging.

Manufacturers can strive to market only nontoxic products to children. When toxic products or related products are marketed (such as false nails for girls, which call for highly toxic false nail adhesive remover), the toxic products should be supplied in child-resistant packaging and should be graphically labeled as toxic.

8.C.9 Mass Media

Targeted messages might foster public awareness of the availability of poison-control centers and of syrup of ipecac and the appropriate use of each, as well as of the most common poisoning hazards for children.

Safe storage of hazardous materials can become the norm in households portrayed on television or in other media.

Self-poisoning is a common method of self-inflicted injury in adolescents who attempt suicide. The role of the media and other forms of mass communication in preventing suicide by children and adolescents is discussed more thoroughly in chapter 14.

References

Caravati, EM, and Litovitz, TL. 1988. Pediatric cyanide intoxication and death from an acetonitrile-containing cosmetic. *JAMA* 260(23):3470.

Consumer Product Safety Commission. 1988. Poison Prevention Packaging Act of 1970. 16 *CFR* 1700.

Consumer Product Safety Commission. 1986. *Poison Prevention Packaging: A Text for Pharmacists and Physicians.* Washington, D.C.: Consumer Product Safety Commission.

Council of State Science Supervisors. 1984. *School Science Laboratories: A Guide to Some Hazardous Substances.* A supplement to NIOSH's *Manual of Safety and Health Hazards in the School Science Laboratory.* Washington, D.C.: Consumer Product Safety Commission.

Edmonson, MB. 1987. Caustic alkali ingestions by farm children. *Pediatrics* 79(3): 413-416.

Farm Safety Association. 1985a. *Manure Gas—Hydrogen Sulphide.* Fact Sheet No. F-006. Guelph, Ontario: Farm Safety Association.

Farm Safety Association. 1985b. *Silo Gas—A Swift and Silent Killer.* Fact Sheet No. F-010. Guelph, Ontario: Farm Safety Association.

Garbarino, J, et al. 1986. *The Psychologically Battered Child.* San Francisco: Jossey-Bass.

Glickman, NW, et al. 1982. Accidental poisoning of children by veterinary drugs. *Natl Clgh Poison Control Cent Bull* 26(2):1-2.

Litovitz, TL. 1988. Lecture presented at Johns Hopkins Hospital, Baltimore, Md., December 9.

Litovitz, TL, et al. 1988. 1987 annual report of the American Association of Poison Control Centers National Data Collection System. *Am J Emerg Med* 6(5): 479-515.

McIntire, MS, and Angle, CR. 1983. Regional poison-control centers improve patient care, editorial. *N Engl J Med* 308(4):219.

Newberger, E, and Hyde, J. 1975. Child abuse: Principles and implications of current pediatric practice. *Pediatr Clin North Am* 22(3):695-715.

Sibert, JR. 1975. Stress in families of children who have ingested poisons. *Br Med J* 3:87.

Thompson, DF, et al. 1983. Evaluation of regional and nonregional poison centers. *N Engl J Med* 308(4):191-194.

Trinkoff, AM, and Baker, SP. 1986. Poisoning hospitalizations and deaths from solids and liquids among children and teenagers. *Am J Public Health* 76(6): 657-660.

Additional Sources of Information

Kresel, JJ, and Lovejoy, FH Jr. 1981. Poisonings and child abuse, in Ellerstein, NS (ed.): *Child Abuse and Neglect: A Medical Reference.* New York: John Wiley and Sons, pp. 307-313.

Rosenberg, D. 1987. Web of deceit: A literature review of Munchausen syndrome by proxy. *Child Abuse Negl* 11:547-563.

American Association of Poison Control Centers (AAPCC)
Arizona Poison and Drug Information Center
Health Science Center
Room 3204K
1501 N. Campbell Hall
Tucson, AZ 85725
602-626-7899
Standards for regional poison-control centers, annual data reports.

Consumer Product Safety Commission (CPSC)
5401 Westbard Avenue
Washington, DC 20207
800-638-CPSC or 301-492-6424
Information on Poison Prevention Packaging Act, general information on childhood poisonings.

Poison Prevention Week Council
PO Box 1543
Washington, DC 20013
Materials for community activities to promote poison prevention.

9

Choking and Suffocation

9.A Facts

Children die when air cannot get in and out of their lungs and consequently no fresh supply of oxygen is available to be carried by the blood to body tissues like the heart and brain. Carbon dioxide levels rise, leading to changes in body chemistry which are quickly life-threatening. This kind of event is called *asphyxiation* or *suffocation*, and the number of ways this catastrophe can happen are described by several sometimes overlapping terms. A child *chokes* when material put into the mouth catches in the throat or passes farther into the airway (trachea and/or bronchi) and obstructs air movement, or when the child sucks (*aspirates*) material into the airway or its branches in the lungs by breathing or gasping. On the other hand, air may be blocked from outside the body, as when a child is caught in an airtight compartment from which the oxygen is gradually depleted by breathing; when airtight material, such as plastic, covers the nose and mouth; when the neck is constricted (*strangulation*); or when the chest is compressed so that breathing is impossible, as in some crush injuries. *Entrapment* (being caught in a position or location and unable to move) may initiate any of these latter events. In some circumstances more than one descriptive term may be used appropriately, but all imply compromise of airflow.

Choking on food or objects, aspirating them into the airway, and suffocation by materials that block the external airway are of special concern in very young children. Choking is a major hazard in the first few years of life. Death rates are especially high in the first few months, when aspiration of feedings or vomit is a problem in frail children. Choking on solid food causes an estimated 75 deaths annually in the under-5 age-group, and choking on nonfood items causes an additional 150 deaths. Many of these deaths should be preventable because the characteristics of commonly involved foods and objects have been identified.

Size, shape, and consistency are major determinants of whether a food or object is apt to block the airway and lead to death. Round foods are especially hazardous, as are foods that are pliable and conform to the airway, or of a size that can obstruct the airway: hot dogs, round candies, nuts, and grapes are the leading culprits in fatal choking. Materials such as peanuts and watermelon seeds may be too small to block the main airway but can be aspirated into the branches in the lungs, with severe consequences.

Similarly, young children are endangered by little balls, pacifiers, squeeze toys or rattles, and balloons (either uninflated, underinflated, or pieces thereof). Pull-tabs from aluminum beverage cans, plastic coating of disposable diapers, pieces of styrofoam from cups, and vinyl or plastic from playpen rails, etc., also present a choking and aspiration hazard. The danger is greatest in children less than 2 years old but is also significant in the 3- to 5-year population and in older children who are developmentally delayed.

Some of these choking hazards have been addressed by the Consumer Product Safety Commission (CPSC), for example, by its specifications for pacifiers sold in the United States, although those purchased elsewhere or makeshift pacifiers (see section 9.C.2) may still be an aspiration hazard.

The CPSC "small-parts" standard bans toys and other products for children under 3 years of age if the products or their detachable components are small enough to fit inside a truncated cylinder that is 1.25 inches (31.7 mm) in diameter with sides that range from 1.0 to 2.25 inches (25.4–57.1 mm) (CPSC 1988a). (Even larger objects, especially if they have rounded edges, can pose a problem.) Toys do not have to meet this standard if the label indicates that they are intended for children aged 3 or older. Unfortunately, labels do not specifically warn purchasers that the toys pose a choking hazard to younger children. As a result, parents may be attracted to them in the belief that they will be stimulating to younger children, or may purchase them for older children without recognizing the danger to younger siblings who have access to the toy (see figure 9–1). Balloons have been exempted from the regulation, although they are the toy most likely to kill a child (Baker and Fisher 1980).

Similarly, manufacturers have not been required to modify foods (e.g., redesign hot dogs so that a bite-size piece does not form a perfect plug) or provide appropriate, unambiguous age-warning labels, such as "Not intended to be given to children under 4 years of age. Fatal choking may result." Few caretakers know that hot dogs, grapes, etc., should not be offered to younger children without at least slicing them lengthwise.

Death rates due to suffocation from obstruction of the nose and mouth or pressure on the throat or chest are highest during the first year of life, when almost 200 infants die annually because someone in the same bed rolls over on them; or their face becomes wedged against or buried in a mattress, pillow, infant cushion, sofa, etc., or is covered by or pressed against a plastic bag. Cribs are a strangulation hazard when the vertical railings are spaced more than $2\frac{3}{8}$ inches apart, when the corner posts extend more than $\frac{1}{16}$ inch above the end panels, when the headboards have cut-out areas that can trap a child's head, when crib hardware is not securely fastened, or when end panels do not extend below the mattress. Cribs can

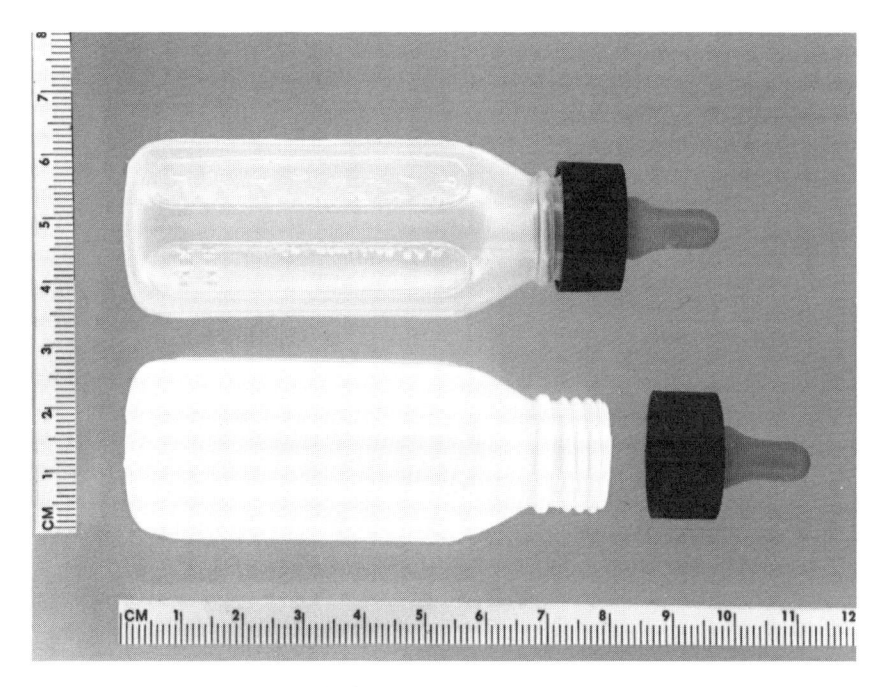

FIGURE 9-1. *Toy bottles with detachable nipples that do not pass small parts test. Package, labeled "Ages 3 and up," has no clear warning that the small parts present a choking hazard for younger children.*

permit suffocation when there is space between the mattress and the side of the crib (an adult should not be able to insert two fingers in the space) (see figure 9-2). The sides of mesh cribs and playpens, if left folded down, form a pocket into which children can become wedged and suffocate. The CPSC has now regulated full-size and non-full-size cribs (CPSC 1988c), but cribs manufactured before the standards took effect are still in use and can endanger children because of widely spaced slats, unsafe corner-post extensions, or gaps between mattress and sides, among other things.

Entrapment of the head with resulting strangulation has occurred with toy boxes whose lids fall down on the child's neck, with folding gates that have large V-shaped upper edges (these gates have now been banned), and with bunk beds which permit a child's body to slip between parts of the frame or between the guardrail and the mattress. Anything that can become wrapped around a child's neck can lead to hanging or ligature strangulation (external pressure on the neck without the body hanging); children have been strangled by drapery cords, crib toys on strings, pacifier cords, restraining devices, or long ribbons on clothing. In older children, scarves and neck strings have sometimes been caught in snowmobiles, engines, or escalators.

Suffocation in abandoned refrigerators, freezers, and other air-sealed containers such as coolers is still a problem, even though household refrig-

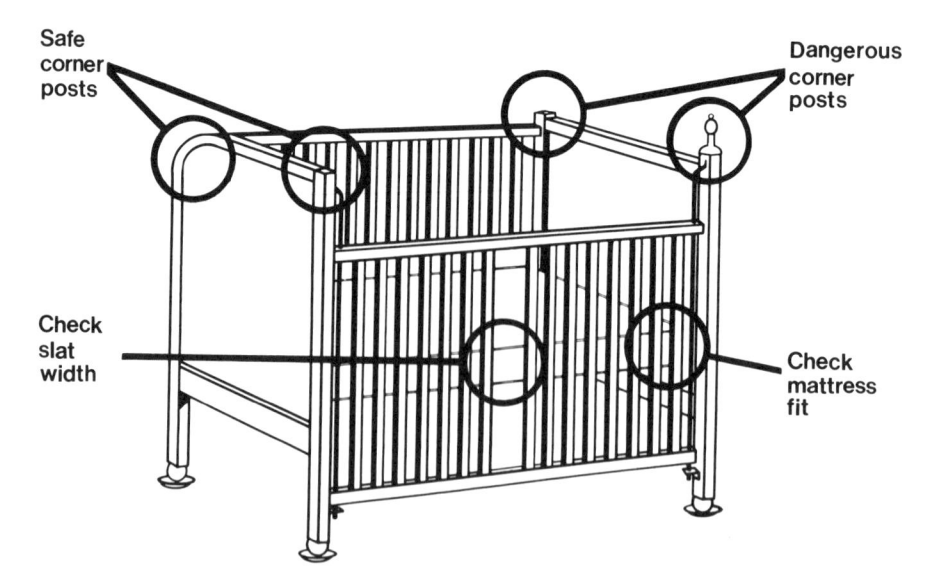

FIGURE 9-2. *Aspects to consider to prevent choking and suffocation hazards in cribs. (Courtesy of the Danny Foundation. Reprinted by permission.)*

erators are now required to have latches which open easily from the inside to enable a child to escape (CPSC 1988b). Boys have much higher suffocation rates than girls; their deaths sometimes result from being trapped when playing with automatic garage doors, in elevators in housing projects or other high-rise buildings, or in trenches and loose dirt where cave-ins can occur. Children on farms are at risk of entrapment and suffocation in grain storage bins and grain transport vehicles (Tevis and Finck 1989).

Some studies estimate that about one-tenth of the suffocation deaths during the first year of life are intentional, that is, inflicted (Emery 1985). The figure may be higher in low-resource, high-stress populations. The need for parental counseling and extra support systems is especially great in the case of mothers with postnatal depression.

In adolescents, intentional hanging is second only to gunshots as a means of committing suicide. About 100 children under 15 years old hang themselves each year.

9.B Developmental Considerations
9.B.1 Infants

Size is a major contributor to choking and suffocation deaths of infants. The infant's head is relatively large compared with its body. The infant's body can slip through narrow spaces, like those between widely spaced crib bars, but the head may be too large to follow. The infant, in effect, hangs.

Infants are not able to extricate themselves from tight places. They may become wedged, for instance, between the mattress and the side of the crib and suffocate. Low-birthweight infants may breathe poorly in standard car safety seats (see section 3.C.2).

The normal and developmentally facilitating tendency of infants to mouth objects places them at special danger. Their airways are small, easily blocked, and difficult to intubate (enter with an endotracheal tube) during emergency resuscitation efforts. In addition, infants may be more likely to be injured by airway rescue efforts, such as abdominal thrusts, than older children.

Infants are particularly vulnerable to inflicted choking and suffocation, being able neither to resist effectively nor to communicate.

9.B.2 Toddlers

For toddlers, all objects are potential playthings. Their tireless interest in exploration, coupled with their often surprising ability to reach, climb, and manipulate, gives them access to a wide range of objects on which to choke and entices them into situations in which they can become entrapped or hang. Many objects which would be inaccessible to the infant or understood to be dangerous by the older child are simultaneously available to and not perceived to be dangerous by the toddler. Furthermore, the airway remains small and easily blocked by unchewed foods and other small, round, hard objects prevalent in the environment.

9.B.3 Preschoolers

As children move through the preschool period, choking and suffocation events reflect the use of more elaborate objects and settings for play. Fantasy is crucial for the healthy development of children of this age. The abandoned refrigerator becomes a ship or tank, the attic trunk a playhouse. The preschooler may not be able to open these from the inside or to signal for help.

9.B.4 and 9.B.5 Elementary School Ages and Young Adolescents

While older children are less likely to choke or aspirate than infants and toddlers, they still are at significant risk for suffocation at their play or work, which is now more oriented toward the "real world." For example, they may be buried in the collapse of tunnels, forts, or clubhouses that they construct or as they trespass to explore a real construction site. They may suffocate in grain bins or gravity wagons as they play or help on the farm.

Older children, especially boys, may knowingly court danger for the thrill of it all. They may be asphyxiated when their airway or their chest is crushed as they race under an automatic garage door or play in an elevator shaft. Early-age suicides may be accomplished by hanging (see section 14.A).

9.C Opportunities for Protection

STRATEGIES FOR PREVENTING CHOKING AND SUFFOCATION
(high-priority strategies are indicated by a △)

Designing Products

    Redesign toys, toy parts, and round manufactured foods to reduce the likelihood of choking and aspiration.

    Design children's furniture to prevent entrapment and strangulation.

    Design car restraints to accommodate low-birthweight children.

    Design gravity boxes for grain transport with rainwater drainage systems that do not require the door to open, or equip doors with safety locks (CDC 1988).

Adding Warning Labels

△ Place warnings on hazardous toys, balloons, peanuts, hot dogs, etc., that specify the danger of choking.

    Place warning decals on all grain storage bins, wagons, and trucks.

Changing the Environment

△ Replace cribs that do not comply with latest CPSC and voluntary standards.

△ Replace automatic garage doors that do not reverse when an object is struck while closing.

    Replace stair gates that have V-shaped upper edges or other parts that can trap heads.

    Remove doors from discarded air-sealed containers, such as refrigerators and freezers.

    Shorten drapery cords or remove from children's reach.

    Fill in spaces between crib and mattress where a child's body could become wedged or slip through.

    Require childproof barriers at excavation sites.

Changing Adult Behavior

    Remove cords from pacifiers, crib toys.

    Slice hot dogs in thin slices lengthwise or avoid giving to young children.

    Substitute low-risk foods for peanuts, flat candies for round candies, etc.

    Provide support system for new mothers likely to experience postnatal depression or to neglect or abuse children.

    Avoid taking infant into adult's bed.

    Don't allow children to enter grain transport equipment or bins with flowing grain.

Improving Emergency Care

△ Train parents, teachers, and caregivers in techniques to expel foreign objects and restore breathing: back blows and chest thrusts for infants, subdiaphragmatic abdominal thrusts for children and adolescents.

Train rural rescue squads in grain bin rescue procedures.

9.C.1 Schools and Child Care Centers

Because children under 3 years of age are most at risk for choking and aspiration incidents, child care centers and day care providers should be especially attentive to choking hazards. The general recommendations apply to all schools, however. Teachers, aides, mealtime and lunchroom personnel, volunteers, and day care providers should be taught what items constitute choking hazards, including small parts of toys. They also should be required to know first aid techniques for airway rescue. First aid posters should be displayed in lunchrooms and other rooms where food is eaten. Hot dogs, nuts, grapes, and other hazardous foods should not be served to young children.

Students should be taught airway rescue techniques as part of a required health, physical education, or other required class no later than grade 8. Home economics, health, child development, or other classes dealing with family management should emphasize home safety and choking hazards. Appropriate foods for children of different developmental stages should be discussed.

Schools and day care centers should establish standards concerning cribs, playpens, baby gates, toy and storage chests, crib toys, and other toys based on the latest voluntary and CPSC standards. Newly purchased items should meet the standards; older items not meeting the standards should be immediately removed from use and discarded or modified. Periodic maintenance checks should be conducted to ensure continued compliance. Schools and child care centers should ask the CPSC to keep them advised of newly discovered or emerging hazards via the CPSC's free publication, *Safety News*. For example, manufacturers recently recalled polystyrene pellet-filled "bean bag" cushions for infants after the CPSC learned of an unusually high number of deaths associated with the relatively new product (CPSC 1990a). Basketlike cots with soft mattresses (Oudesluys-Murphy and van Yperen 1988) and waterbeds (CPSC 1989a) may also present suffocation hazards.

Where infants and small children are involved, drapery or shade cords should be cleated or fastened and clothes lines should be out of children's reach or removed. Child care policy manuals should outline procedures for storage and disposal of plastic bags, plastic wrap, and disposable diapers. Disposable plastic diapers have been involved in choking and suffocation incidents; they should be covered with clothing at all times (Johnson 1986). School policy should state that pacifiers are not to be tied to clothing or worn around the neck. Teachers and day care providers should discuss these and other choking hazards, for example, inappropriate jewelry, toys, or foods brought from home, with parents.

School policy should state that balloons are not allowed as classroom or party decorations for young children. Peanuts and other small, round objects such as jelly beans should not be used for party games or favors. Those working with older children should be aware of choking hazards of scarves, jewelry, and loose or baggy clothing (ASBO 1986) when using power tools (e.g., shop and home economics classes). Schools should establish and enforce suitable safety practices. The danger of flowing grain entrapment and suffocation should be discussed in agriculture classes.

All schools and child care facilities should require playground equipment, indoor play gyms, and all banisters and railings to comply with CPSC guidelines to prevent head entrapment. (See additional sources of information; guidelines are discussed further in chapter 15.)

Crawl spaces and other confined areas should be locked so that young children cannot enter them (CAPFA 1987). Appliances such as freezers, washers, dryers, and coolers and other storage chests should be in a locked area inaccessible to children. Fences or barriers should be erected to prevent children from playing in areas of possible cave-ins, such as excavation, mining, and construction sites on or near school property.

9.C.2 Health Care Providers

The recommended first aid procedures for the very young choking child have recently been revised (AAP 1988; AHA 1988). Further revisions are possible. The health care provider should keep abreast of the recommendations published by the American Academy of Pediatrics Committee on Accident and Poison Prevention in the journal *Pediatrics*.

Parents may be largely unaware of choking and suffocation hazards. The best time to address suffocation hazards presented by nursery equipment may be the prenatal visit or class, when purchasing decisions are still to be made. It is particularly important to address at early visits the question of where the baby will be or is sleeping (see section 9.A). Some low-birthweight infants cannot breathe properly in a standard car seat (they are subject to "postural" strangulation); health care providers can instruct parents in proper fitting techniques (see section 3.C.2).

Nutrition guidance should include advice about food size and consistency appropriate for developmental age. Since most severe choking events which involve food in childhood occur in the earliest years and involve round, hard foods, these are to be avoided. Specifically to be prohibited because of their association with fatal chokings in young children are hot dogs which have not been sliced lengthwise and cut into small pieces, peanuts, grapes, and hard candies.

Current disease-coding practices fail to distinguish between asphyxiation caused by direct entry of food into the airway and food refluxing into the airway from the stomach. Changes in the coding would make study of the causes of asphyxiation more straightforward.

Nonfood objects of many different types are also associated with airway obstruction (see section 9.A). The health care provider should counsel about the dangers of access to small objects, about the need to avoid toys with small parts for a child under 3 even though a parent believes the child precocious, about the desirability of supervision and the currently recommended techniques of first aid for choking children of different ages. In addition, the health care provider should be an informed source of information about the particular risks of suffocation or strangulation associated with children's products and automatic garage doors, as well as in flowing grain or under gravity wagon doors in rural areas.

Recalls are frequently announced when asphyxiation is reported with product use. Health care sites should have a prominent and consistent place to post such notices. If the practice produces a newsletter for patients, recall notices might be included. Health care providers should also report product-related asphyxiation incidents to the CPSC (see additional sources of information).

Children are exposed to choking, strangulation, and suffocation hazards in many hospitals (Banco and Powers 1988). Pedestal-style electric beds with "walk-away" down controls have caused entrapment deaths (Merz 1983) and should not be used on pediatric wards. "Makeshift" pacifiers constructed of two-piece nursing bottle nipples should never be used (Millunchick and McArtor 1986). Not only does such a practice present a direct hazard at the time, it also encourages the baby to refuse other safer pacifiers and the parent to continue to rely on the makeshift device.

The cause of some acute life-threatening events (ALTEs) and some unexplained asphyxiations in infancy is deliberate suffocation of the infant by a caregiver. Certainly, most asphyxiations are not due to child abuse. In most cases the role of the health care provider will be to reassure the grieving or worried parents and not to add the burden of suspicion to their problems. However, the health care provider should not ignore the fact that infants are sometimes deliberately smothered. Such acts produce characteristic patterns on multichannel physiological recording equipment used to monitor infants (Southall et al. 1987). While a diagnosis of fatal child abuse occurs too late to prevent injury to the smothered child, it may protect future children.

Health care providers serving young adolescents should be aware of the warning signs of suicide, which may be accomplished by hanging (see chapter 14).

9.C.3 Public Agencies

Social-service agencies should have a routine protocol for identifying and remedying the principal choking, aspiration, and suffocation risks. An inspection should be carried out at the homes of children at special risk and at all foster care homes. Deliberate suffocation is a common form of infanticide. Social-service workers should concentrate on helping new mothers prepare for and deal with postnatal depression in cases where abuse or neglect is suspected in previous poorly explained infant deaths.

Local and regional building codes should require safe spacing between stair rails. The 6-inch spacing currently allowed by many codes is wide enough that 95% of all children under 10 years old can slip through (Meyer 1990), thereby permitting strangulation by hanging. A 4-inch spacing requirement, which has been adopted by several model codes, is preferable.

Public agencies should require that discarded refrigerators, freezers, washers, dryers, and coolers have the doors removed, and that construction sites be fenced off so children can't enter. These regulations should be strictly enforced. Agencies working with farm families can require or distribute warning signs for grain wagons and bins and can teach children in farm safety classes about the suffocation hazards.

9.C.4 Legislators and Regulators

The CPSC "small-parts" toy regulation (CPSC 1988a) has been called inadequate in several ways, including the age-group covered and the test fixture used, which screens out objects small enough to enter the lower throat and trachea but fails to identify objects which can enter the mouth and obstruct the airway at the level of the back of the mouth and upper throat (CPSC 1989b). The CPSC has announced its intention to keep the current test fixture but to address choking hazards for children older than 3 and to consider regulations for balloons, small balls, and marbles, which are exempt from current regulation. Regulations should be improved for toy design, and toy labeling should be regulated, particularly with regards to telling parents about the specific hazard involved. Surveys of adults have shown that the current format of age labeling (e.g., "Recommended for ages 3 and up") is often misunderstood. Some think that it refers to the ability or interest level of the child, instead of properly perceiving this as a choking-hazard warning. Age-labeling regulation should be redrawn to ensure a greater level of consumer understanding.

The voluntary industry standards on crib toys also have been found to be inadequate; the length requirement for cords used to attach toys to cribs, to suspend toys, or to activate parts of toys is unfounded, and the standard requires a label recommending that parents remove the toy just when the toy would be of most use to the child developmentally (CPSC 1987a).

Despite regulations introduced in 1974 and subsequently strengthened by amendment to address neck entrapment and by voluntary standards to upgrade structural integrity, one study (Kraus 1985) found no significant reduction in strangulation crib deaths, although a CPSC report claims that the 1974 standard on crib-slat widths brought about a 40% reduction in injuries and deaths (Kraus 1985). Because of the long life of cribs, the regulation may require more time to be evidently effective in reducing fatalities. A revision to the voluntary standard currently being adopted, which limits corner-post extensions to $\frac{1}{16}$ inch from $\frac{5}{8}$ inch, may further reduce fatalities.

Regulations governing refrigerator and freezer design (CPSC 1988b) seem to have been effective in reducing the number of entrapment deaths involving these appliances. Researchers have pointed out, however, that the minimum of 15 pounds of internal pressure specified by the standard to open the door was not within the capability of a significant number of children tested (Kraus 1985). Children suffocate because of entrapment in other devices as well, such as dryers, washers, portable coolers, and refrigerators in campers. Regulations could be introduced to prevent entrapment in any air-sealed storage unit (Kraus 1985).

Regulators could reduce the use of suffocating plastics by calling for more porous or less static plastics (Kraus 1985) or the use of nonsuffocating materials.

Local legislators should consider ordinances requiring protective barriers to prevent children from playing near sites of possible cave-ins of earth or sand, such as construction sites.

9.C.5 Law Enforcement Professionals

Smothering an infant leaves little or no physical evidence of trauma (Zumwalt and Hirsch 1980). Because deaths due to intentional asphyxiation may be difficult to detect, law enforcement officers need to be appropriately alert to suspicious signs, such as superficial abrasions around the nose, lips, and gums (Zumwalt and Hirsch 1980). Careful observations can be made while maintaining appropriate sensitivity to the feelings of parents in a crisis. Judgments can be postponed until later, when time has permitted the sorting out of evidence.

Police in England have aided child-protection cases by covert video surveillance in hospitals of parents whose infants have suffered repeated mysterious spells and who are suspected of intentional suffocation (Southall et al. 1987). With concrete video evidence, medical staff avoided confronting parents with possibly incorrect suspicions or accusations while still protecting the child. Such surveillance in the United States would raise currently unanswered questions of constitutional law.

9.C.6 Voluntary Organizations

The role for voluntary organizations in preventing childhood choking appears limited at this time. Certainly, groups sponsoring functions which include small children should avoid providing decorations, foods, or favors on which children might choke. Groups whose activities include child care should be certain that facilities, equipment, and toys are free of choking and suffocation hazards. Community groups might monitor solid waste disposal in their area to make certain that doors are removed from abandoned appliances such as refrigerators and freezers and also monitor construction sites to be certain access to excavations is barred.

4-H clubs and other groups that serve children in rural areas can work to educate children and parents about the suffocation dangers involved when working with flowing grain or playing in empty gravity boxes. Groups can help distribute warning decals to be placed on grain storage bins and wagons.

9.C.7 Designers, Architects, Builders, and Engineers

Toys with small parts are currently labeled as "not intended for children younger than 3," "ages 3 and up," or similarly. Evidence suggests that such labeling does not provide parents with the clear message that the young child may mouth the toy and choke. There is room for improvement in labeling. The current test cylinder used to gauge whether an object will block a child's airway may not be ideal (see section 9.C.4).

Asphyxiation hazards for the children who will use or misuse products or be exposed to them through adult use should be considered when new products are designed. Otolaryngological consultation is useful. The review of previous experience may decrease the hazard with future designs. Products of recent or current concern because they have been associated with choking, aspiration, strangulation, or suffocation include furniture and products designed for babies (cribs, pellet-filled infant cushions, high chairs, playpens, accordian-style baby gates, retracting car seat straps, ladders on toy slides, crib toys), button batteries, plastic buttons from gift-wrapping bows, pull-tabs from aluminum beverage cans, small projectiles from toys, toy-box lids which can close on the child's neck, styrofoam cups, collapsible washing lines, plastic bags, large appliances, sofa beds, bunk beds, and recliners. Existing products can be modified to reduce the hazard; for example, dry cleaners' bags could have ventilating holes, bow pins have been redesigned, new refrigerator doors can be opened with little force from the inside, swimming pool drainage pipes can be made too small for a child to fit in and can be covered with nonremovable grates (see chapter 17). Adherence to CPSC playground guidelines should reduce hangings through entanglement of head or clothing (see additional sources of information). The top bunks of bunk beds should have guardrails on all four sides to prevent falls, but the gap between the lower edge of the guardrails and the upper edge of the bed frame should not be more than $3\frac{1}{2}$ inches. Larger spaces permit entrapment and strangulation. Likewise, cross ties must be securely attached to the frame to support the mattress, in order to prevent entrapment from collapse (CPSC 1987).

Coins, commonly mouthed by children, may become lodged in the airway or the gastrointestinal tract. They should continue to be minted in such a fashion that they are radiopaque and therefore easily identified during radiologic evaluation. Other small objects, including barrettes and toy parts, should also be radiopaque. Automatic garage doors need to stop and reverse when an object is encountered during closing; all garage door openers should meet at least the ANSI/UL 1982 voluntary standard. Periodic testing and maintenance even of doors that were manufactured in compliance with that standard is required (CPSC 1990b). Elevator doors must be closed with a mechanism which children cannot subvert to gain access to the shaft.

Some small, prematurely born infants appear not able to maintain an airway when strapped into currently marketed car safety seats. They develop dangerously low blood oxygen levels. New designs are needed for these small infants, or, ideally, current designs should be modified to be useful for infants of any size and developmental stage (see section 3.C.2).

Window coverings (draperies, blinds) should be designed to open and close without a long loop of cord. Children inadvertently hang themselves in window-covering cords. Brackets or other convenient and attractive means of storing excess cord out of children's reach should be provided with the coverings.

9.C.8 Business and Industry

Food products produced specifically for young children should not be hard or pliable and round and the size of the airway. Flight attendants should not offer peanuts to children; in fact, they should replace peanuts with some other type of snack such as small crackers or pretzels that are unlikely to cause aspiration or fatal choking.

Consistently used, uniform, improved warning labels should be developed for food, toys, and other items children might choke on. Labels should specify the hazard involved—for example, "fatal choking can result." Diaper services and infant-product manufacturers should be required to use only nonsuffocating materials for bags and packaging.

Products which are reported to be associated with choking, aspiration, strangulation, and suffocation should be promptly and voluntarily removed from the market. Such cooperation decreases a company's exposure to liability. Rigorous and responsive voluntary industry standards obviate the need for new regulations which historically have been tedious and delayed. Manufacturers can recall or offer rebates for products associated with asphyxiation that were made before standards applied, such as cribs. Premarket testing of toys and children's products for safety can prevent injuries and deaths. Toys, cribs, and other products imported from foreign countries may be in violation of U.S. mandatory and voluntary standards. Manufacturers and importers must be aware of and comply with all pertinent standards.

9.C.9 Mass Media

Awareness of choking, aspiration, strangulation, and suffocation hazards can be increased by ample coverage. Many materials children choke on, such as balloons, hot dogs, and peanuts, are so commonly given to children that their hazardous qualities are unrecognized or ignored presently. Reminders are needed. Products designed for infants and young children that have caused asphyxiation deaths are often recalled. The news media provide the most ready access many consumers have to this recall information.

In addition to targeting the adult population, the mass media could produce public-service announcements for integration into children's programming. These messages could teach the dangers of plastic bags, discarded appliances with doors, tunneling, and a variety of other stunts that might lead to choking, strangulation, or suffocation.

Airway rescue techniques (such as abdominal thrusts for children and back blows and chest thrusts for infants) are easily demonstrated and quite visual; they need wide dissemination.

References

American Academy of Pediatrics. 1988. First aid for the choking child, policy statement. *Pediatrics* 81(5):740.
American Heart Association. 1988. *Textbook of Pediatric Basic Life Support*. Dallas: American Heart Association.
Association of School Business Officials International. 1986. *School Safety Handbook*, revised version. Reston, Va.: Association of School Business Officials.
Baker, SP, and Fisher, RS. 1980. Childhood asphyxiation by choking or suffocation. *JAMA* 244:1343.
Banco, L, and Powers, A. 1988. Hospitals: Unsafe environments for children. *Pediatrics* 82(5):794–797.
Centers for Disease Control. 1988. *Farm-related injury deaths among young children—Wisconsin and Illinois*. EPI 86-70-2. Atlanta: Centers for Disease Control.
Child Accident Prevention Foundation of Australia. 1987. *Guidelines on Safety in Family Day Care Homes*. Melbourne, Australia: Child Accident Prevention Foundation of Australia.
Consumer Product Safety Commission. 1987a. *Human Factors Evaluation of Provisions which Address Crib Toy Strangulations in the Toy Safety Voluntary Standard*. Report prepared by SW Deppa. Washington, D.C.: Consumer Product Safety Commission.
Consumer Product Safety Commission. 1987b. *Bunk Beds*. Product Safety Fact Sheet 71. Washington, D.C.: Consumer Product Safety Commission.
Consumer Product Safety Commission. 1988a. Method for identifying toys and other articles intended for use by children under 3 years of age which present choking, aspiration, or ingestion hazards because of small parts. 16 *CFR* 1501.
Consumer Product Safety Commission. 1988b. Refrigerator safety act regulations. 16 *CFR* 1750.
Consumer Product Safety Commission. 1988c. Requirements for full-size baby cribs and Requirements for non-full-size baby cribs. 16 *CFR* 1508 and 1509.
Consumer Product Safety Commission. 1989a. Infants should not be left on adult or youth beds. *Safety News* December.

Consumer Product Safety Commission. 1989b. *A Physiological Review of Toys Causing Choking in Children.* Report prepared by S Pepper. Washington, D.C.: Consumer Product Safety Commission.

Consumer Product Safety Commission. 1990a. Jumping-Jacks Shoes Inc. recalls "Baby Jacks" infant cushions because of suffocation risk. *Safety News* May.

Consumer Product Safety Commission. 1990b. Parents urged to replace unsafe garage doors. *Safety News* April.

Emery, JL. 1985. Infanticide, filicide, and cot death. *Arch Dis Child* 60:505-507.

Johnson, CM. 1986. Disposable plastic diapers: A foreign body hazard. *Otolaryngol Head Neck Surg* 94(2):235-236.

Kraus, JF. 1985. Effectiveness of measures to prevent unintentional deaths of infants and children from suffocation and strangulation. *Public Health Rep* 100(2):231-240.

Merz, B. 1983. Hospital-bed deaths, injuries force down-switch modifications. *JAMA* 250(7):871-872.

Meyer, W. 1990. NEAT File: Codes and standards of care. *Architecture* January.

Millunchick, EW, and McArtor, RD. 1986. Fatal aspiration of a makeshift pacifier. *Pediatrics* 77(3):369-370.

Oudesluys-Murphy, AM, and van Yperen, WJ. 1988. The cot in cot deaths. *Eur J Pediatr* 147(1):85-86.

Southall, DP, et al. 1987. Apnoeic episodes induced by smothering: Two cases identified by covert video surveillance. *Br Med J Clin Res* 294(6588):1637-1641.

Tevis, C, and Finck, C. 1989. We kill too many farm kids, special report. *Successful Farming* Mid-February.

Zumwalt, RE, and Hirsch, CS. 1980. Subtle fatal child abuse. *Hum Pathol* 11(2):167-174.

Additional Sources of Information

American Heart Association (AHA)
National Center
7320 Greenville Avenue
Dallas, TX 75231
214-706-1360
   Information on Pediatric Basic Life Support classes.

American Red Cross (ARC)
2025 E Street, NW
Washington, DC 20006
202-728-6531
   Information on CPR classes.

Americans for Democratic Action (ADA)
511 K Street, NW
Washington, DC 20005
202-638-6447
   Annual toy safety report.

Consumer Product Safety Commission (CPSC)
5401 Westbard Avenue
Washington, DC 20207
800-638-CPSC or 301-492-6424
   Free publication, *Safety News*, lists CPSC and manufacturers' warnings and recalls; information on crib, nursery, and toy safety, and *A Handbook for Public Playground Safety*, volumes 1 and 2.

The Danny Foundation
PO Box 680
Alamo, CA 94507
800-83DANNY
   Educational materials on safe cribs.

Farm Safety Association
340 Woodlawn Road, Suite 22
Guelph, Ontario N1H 7K6
Canada
519-823-5600
   Information on flowing grain entrapment and rescue techniques.

Farm Safety for Just Kids
716 Main Street
PO Box 458
Earlham, IA 50072
515-758-2827
   Educational materials on suffocation hazards of grain wagons and other farm equipment, warning decals for grain wagons.

Network for Injury Prevention in
   Buildings (NIP)
Box 67, Blue Ridge Hospital
University of Virginia Medical Center
Charlottesville, VA 22901
804-924-5308
   Information on building codes.

Society for Automotive Engineers
400 Commonwealth Drive
Warrendale, PA 15096
412-776-4841
   Information on anthropometry (publishes and sells *Anthropometry of Infants, Children, and Youths to Age 18 for Product Safety Design* by RG Synder et al.).

Toys to Grow On
PO Box 17
Long Beach, CA 90801
213-603-8890
   No-Choke Testing Tube (similar to CPSC small-parts test fixture).

10

Falls

10.A Facts

Falls are the leading cause of nonfatal injury. In children they account for about one-third of emergency department visits for injury and 35% of hospital admissions for head injury. Although the number of deaths is much lower than for deaths related to motor vehicles, drowning, or house fires, nearly 200 children aged 0-14 die each year as the result of falls. Death rates are especially high in Asian and black children and in urban areas. The highest death rate is seen during the first year of life.

Falls occur under a wide variety of circumstances, but the risk of death or permanent impairment is strongly related to the height of the fall and the nature of the material struck. Falls from windows, a serious problem in the summertime among children younger than 5, increase in their severity as the height of the window and the hardness of the surface increase. From second-story windows, for example, falls usually are not fatal unless the child lands on concrete. Falls from playground equipment are discussed in chapter 15.

Many falls take place from children's furniture. Each year some 9,000 injuries are related to cribs, 8,000 to high chairs, and 22,000 to bunk beds. For each of these products, the majority of injuries are caused by falls.

Most falls down stairs do not have serious consequences (Joffe and Ludwig 1988), largely because the fall is broken by each step the child lands on. In contrast, when an infant in a baby walker falls down the stairs, the fall may be largely unbroken until the bottom; death or permanent brain injury can result, especially if the floor is concrete, as in many basements. Many of the serious childhood injuries occurring on stairs are related to walkers. A Canadian study found that 42% of all head injuries in children younger than 1 involved walkers and stairs (Stoffman et al. 1984). Since walkers are of no known developmental benefit, their use should be discouraged.

In the case of falls on the same level, sharp corners on furniture, glass coffee tables, and broken glass in play areas are important sources of injury. A 70% reduction in lacerations from broken glass out of doors was noted in a pediatric emergency department after the state passed a "bottle bill" requiring a deposit on glass beverage bottles (Baker et al. 1986).

Other countermeasures shown to be effective include the "Children Can't Fly" program in New York City, in which easily installed window guards were supplied to families with young children living in high-rise buildings (Spiegel and Lindaman 1977).

Intentionally inflicted injuries are sometimes alleged to have resulted from falls. The characteristic patterns of abusive injuries and injuries from falls differ, and medical personnel should be trained in their recognition (Wissow and Wilson 1988). For example, severe or multiple injuries or rib fractures seldom result when a child falls down stairs or from a bed or chair; therefore, reports of such injury events should be carefully investigated.

10.B Developmental Considerations

10.B.1 Infants

For no injury event is the influence of development more apparent than for falls, though falls are common at every age. The infant is often placed at an elevation to be at a convenient height for an adult caregiver, for example, on a changing table, in a crib, on the counter, on an examining table, in a high chair. On elevated surfaces, just as on lower ones, infants roll, scoot, and crawl. If there is no barrier or restraint, they fall.

Parents often fail to anticipate the infant's increasing ability to move. The very first rollover may carry the unguarded infant off furniture onto the floor below. Though it appears that infants begin to recognize drop-offs in the first year of life, they are apparently unable to reliably interpret them or defend against them, for many falls from high surfaces occur.

Because young infants must be carried wherever they go, they can be injured when adults carrying them fall. Home stairways are particularly likely places for adults to fall, and the risk may be increased when the infant blocks the adult's view or limits access to a handrail.

The drive to explore exposes the older infant to the danger of falling even before walking. All children "cruise," that is, walk holding onto hands or furniture, before they walk unassisted. Unstable structures that are easy to grasp contribute to falls (and sometimes crush injuries) at this stage. Many infants crawl up stairs or climb onto chairs before they walk. Falls down stairs are common and falls down stairs in walkers are particularly likely to result in injury.

Infants are, of course, unable to report the circumstances that lead to injury, so inflicted injury (child abuse) is sometimes misrepresented by the caregiver as having resulted from an "accidental" fall.

10.B.2 Toddlers

The child just beginning to walk will fall at the least provocation; making turns, negotiating a threshold, and stooping are impossible. The very term *toddler* speaks to the wide-legged, unsteady walking pattern characteristic of this age. Falls are often to a diaper-padded "sitting" position and damage only pride. However, if the child's body encounters angular, hard surfaces (such as the corner of a coffee table) on the way down, the body may be damaged, too. The impossibility of constant parental vigilance as the major injury-control strategy becomes obvious.

Toddlers dislike being restrained. They do their best to subvert it by wiggling free, climbing out, squiggling under. Devices to prevent falls, such as crib sides, high-chair straps, and stair gates, must be designed with careful attention to such behavior.

Toddlers, often avid climbers busy exploring their world without the aid of experience, are particularly prone to fall from heights because their climbing ability is not matched by balancing or reasoning ability. Their small bodies can slip between widely spaced guardrail uprights, sometimes trapping the head, or their climbing abilities may allow them to fall over the top if they can gain a foothold. These falls—from windows, off high furniture, down stairs in walkers—can cause serious or fatal injury, often of the head. While persons of all ages fall down stairs, children younger than 4 are more likely to suffer head injury than are older children (Joffe and Ludwig 1988).

10.B.3 Preschoolers

By the time children have reached preschool age, they walk and run well and are less closely supervised than infants and toddlers. They are likely to be active outside the home, and their fall injury patterns reflect this, with falls from playground equipment (see chapter 15) and on outside surfaces more prominent. Falls from windows still occur, particularly among boys, as do falls from fire escapes during play.

10.B.4 Elementary School Ages

Older children spend more and more time out of the home and in the company of other children. Injuries may occur as a result of falls from playground equipment (see chapter 15), from a rock pile, down an elevator shaft, on a construction site, or from a rooftop or motor vehicle. Many falls involve recreational products such as bicycles (see chapter 6), roller skates, skateboards, and other sports equipment (see chapter 16), reflecting how children of this age play.

10.B.5 Young Adolescents

Young adolescents, too, fall from heights in diverse locations outside the home, in situations likely to reflect risk-taking behavior in the context of recreational activities. To what extent young adolescents express suicidal intent by jumping from heights is not known.

10.C Opportunities for Protection

> STRATEGIES FOR PREVENTING INJURIES FROM FALLS
> (high-priority strategies are indicated by a △)
>
> *Preventing Access to Heights*
>
> > Avoid infant walkers or use only if they are too wide to go through a door frame or down stairs, or remove wheels.
> >
> > Use cribs with mattresses that can be lowered as the child grows tall and agile enough to climb out.
> >
> > Restrict access to elevator shafts, etc., where older children may be tempted to play.
> >
> > Position fixed ladders on farm structures out of young children's reach or fit with a special barrier. Store portable ladders out of young children's reach and away from hazardous areas such as silos.
>
> *Changing Likely Impact Surfaces*
>
> △ Install padded carpet or other energy-absorbing surface at the foot of stairs, including basement stairs.
>
> > Avoid use of glass coffee tables and other furniture with sharp edges and corners.
> >
> > Use safety glazing on windows and glass doors near children's play areas.
> >
> > Replace concrete and asphalt under playground equipment with materials that absorb more energy.
> >
> > Plant shrubbery or flower beds beneath windows.
> >
> > Keep play surfaces free of broken glass.
>
> *Reducing the Likelihood of Falls*
>
> △ Provide grills or child-resistant screens on upstairs windows.
>
> △ Build stairways with steps that are easily seen, treads large enough to provide adequate footing, and graspable handrails.
>
> △ Build guardrails that small children cannot climb over or fall through.
>
> > Use side rails on bunk beds.
> >
> > Use tip-resistant high chairs with wide bases or replace with low feeding tables.
> >
> > Never leave infant alone on a bed or other unguarded elevated surface.
> >
> > Provide skid-resistant floors and other walking surfaces.

10.C.1 Schools and Child Care Centers

School and child care center personnel can determine where fall injuries are occurring and initiate changes in those areas. Because stairways are a common site for fall injuries, they should be designed not only to be structurally sound but also to help the user perceive the physical characteristics of the stairs easily, by means of visual or tactile cues (Archea et al. 1979) (see section 10.C.7).

Stairways and elevated play areas should have sturdy guardrails of adequate height to prevent falls. These railings should not permit passage of the body or head entrapment. Stair handrails should be present, in good repair, and easy to grasp (see section 10.C.7).

Windows should have screens or guards that limit openings to 4 inches to prevent falls. Windows and glass doors should not be located at the bottom of stairs or in areas likely to be slippery (kitchen areas, locker rooms, and bathrooms) (Clark and Webber 1982). Windows and glass doors adjacent to play areas or otherwise accessible to preschoolers should have safety glazing, such as Plexiglas, or be protected from breaking by guards. Children under 5 years are vulnerable near glass that is less than 1 meter (39 inches) from the floor (Clark and Webber 1982).

Floors should be even and free of tripping hazards. Easy-care carpeting is preferable in day care facilities except in areas for cooking, eating, or toileting (AAP 1987). Energy-absorbing, slip-resistant flooring is ideal for schools. Areas likely to be wet and slippery should have special flooring to provide traction and prevent falls.

Stages and temporary constructions which must support people (stairs, ramps, etc.) should be soundly constructed and regularly inspected. Platforms or ramps more than 30 inches above the ground or floor should have guardrails on all open sides. Stairway or passageway lights should be illuminated whenever the area is in use, and student use of ladders should be supervised (ASBO 1986).

Bleachers are used in many schools, but present design, construction, operation, and maintenance produce hazards not only for fall injury but also for collapse and crush injury (CPSC 1989). Additional attention to this common piece of equipment—including not only changes in the design of new systems but also plans for replacement or improvement of old—is urgently needed.

In schools, the likelihood of tripping or slipping in certain high-activity areas, such as gymnasiums, is clearly foreseeable. In such areas, the walls should be padded or, at the very least, protrusions from the walls should be removed or guarded.

Outdoor hazards, such as hills dropping off to busy roads or pavement, well holes, or sunken windows, should be protected and regularly inspected. Fences and railings should be constructed to discourage climbing; fences should be at the top of a hill if possible, rather than at the bottom, where injuries could result to children sledding, rolling, or riding bikes. Energy-absorbing surfacing can be provided at the bottom of fences, retaining walls (CMHC 1981), and trees (CAPFA 1987).

Fall hazards should be considered in routine safety inspections by child care staff. In addition to those mentioned earlier, hazards include changing tables with no lip or rail on the outside edge; strollers and high chairs with narrow bases, poor construction, or ineffective safety restraints; and cribs with inadequate fastening hardware, mattress bases that do not drop to a position low enough to prevent older infants from climbing out, or containing pillows or toys that enable children to climb out. Adequate storage space should be available so that toys, boots, etc., can be stored out of the line of traffic to prevent tripping. Many falls occur from playground equipment (see chapter 15).

Walkers, which enable very young children to be mobile before they can adequately perceive and avoid dangers, are involved in many childhood injuries. Walkers should not be used, especially in areas where young children can move onto stairs.

10.C.2 Health Care Providers

Health care providers are an important (but not exclusive) source of information for parents about child care equipment and practices and about stages of motor development which may put the child at risk of falling. Child care equipment such as changing tables, cribs, and high chairs should be in good repair, and the restraining devices (belts, straps, and barriers) should be used. For instance, proper use of the high chair includes not only containing the child with the tray, but also fastening a T-shaped strap which goes between the child's legs. Even so, the child should not be left unattended. The parent should be reminded well before the child is likely to pull to standing that the crib mattress should be in its lowest position and then, before the child is likely to be able to climb out, of the need to move the child from the crib to a bed close to the floor. Since the height from which a child falls and the hardness of the surface which the child strikes are important determinants of injury, health care providers might become much more active advocates for changes in caregiving practices and in the design of infant furniture so infants are handled at a lower height and over floors with carpeting and energy-absorbing underpads.

Given the unusual prominence of serious walker-related injury and the absence of any proven developmental advantage to the devices, health care providers may strongly advise against their use. Such advice should be provided at a very early age (probably by the 2-month visit), when parents are not likely to have obtained a walker. If the parent decides against medical advice to use a walker, the health care provider should recommend that guards or gates be used at the head of all stairs (see section 10.C.7) and that the basement door, which often leads down to a concrete floor, be kept secured in such a way that the walker (or the unaccompanied infant or toddler) cannot pass through.

Health care providers should set a good example on their own premises. For instance, infant scales should have appropriate guards, infants should not be left on examining tables, hospital high chairs should be used with restraints, and hospital cafeterias should be equipped with appropriate seating for small children.

Falls are a common reason given for abusive injuries to infants and toddlers. When a seriously injured infant or toddler presents for care and the explanation given is such a fall, inflicted injury (child abuse) should be considered. Studies suggest that injuries sustained from falling the distance from a crib, bed, or sofa to the floor are rarely serious (Nimityongskul and Anderson 1987; Helfer et al. 1977); thus, suspicion should be high when serious injury is attributed to such falls. Intentional injury or purposeful neglect should also be considered even when children fall or are said to have fallen from greater heights.

10.C.3 Public Agencies

Federal, state, and municipal facilities, indoor and outdoor, should be designed to prevent falls (see section 10.C.7). Community planners can see that hazardous areas, natural or man-made, are protected by barriers, guardrails, handrails, and energy-absorbing materials to prevent children and others from fall injuries. Children should be provided with areas to ride bikes and skateboards away from the hazards of traffic. Playgrounds, common sites of falls, are discussed in chapter 15.

Agencies should have routine protocols for inspecting child care facilities and foster homes for fall-related hazards, such as unprotected stairways, walkers, unguarded windows, and unprotected glass. Protective-service workers should be aware that severe injuries rarely result when children fall from couches, beds, or stairs, and should consider whether severe injuries so attributed might have been intentionally inflicted.

Health departments have been effective in preventing falls and reducing injuries by advocating, providing, and requiring inexpensive window guards in apartments where children 10 years or younger reside (Spiegel and Lindaman 1977). Housing codes and inspection procedures should require fall-prevention provisions such as window guards and stairways with adequate lighting.

Snow and ice on streets and sidewalks are related to an increased incidence of falls (Ralis et al. 1988). Provisions for speedy clearance, particularly on school routes, are needed to reduce injury.

10.C.4 Legislators and Regulators

Child-restraint and seat belt legislation not only helps prevent collision injuries but also helps prevent injuries due to falls in or from automobiles. Legislation to prohibit passengers from riding on the exterior of a vehicle, including in the back of a pickup truck, could further reduce fall injuries from motor vehicles (Williams and Goins 1981).

Windows should be required to be screened or otherwise guarded. Baby walkers might also be regulated more thoroughly than the current mandatory regulation, which concerns pinch points only (CPSC 1988). For instance, a Canadian regulation in draft form calls for labeling, tip tests, finger safeguards, a frame size that will not fit through a standard door, and designs which prevent speeds of more than 1 meter/second on a 12-degree incline (James 1988). Closer regulation of other products associated with childhood falls—for example, bunk beds, high chairs, playground equipment, and bathtubs—would be likely to be beneficial. Legislation requiring a deposit on glass beverage bottles ("bottle bills") may help to prevent injuries due to falls onto broken glass (Baker et al. 1986).

10.C.5 Law Enforcement Professionals

Law enforcement officers are often called first to fall injury scenes and should be adequately trained to investigate cases where intentional injury or suicide is suspected. Quite often photographs or field sketches documenting the location of the fall are useful in determining the cause or identifying the mechanism of injury.

Law enforcement personnel should note and report sites that contain fall hazards where children are known to play, such as abandoned buildings, parking garages, and elevator shafts. When possible, they should take action to remove or reduce the hazard. Similarly, the site of inadvertent falls may come to the attention of the police or other law enforcement officers, who then have an opportunity to press for modification of the hazard.

10.C.6 Voluntary Organizations

Voluntary organizations can help to prevent childhood injuries from falls both in and out of the home. Installing window guards on upper-story windows could be a service project, as could monitoring for building repair needs or "attractive nuisances" like abandoned buildings or junk piles from which children might fall during play. Certainly, community buildings that serve children should have appropriate barriers on upper-story windows, and heights on public grounds should have guardrails that are difficult to climb (see section 10.C.7). Playgrounds, the sites of many falls, may be constructed or maintained by community groups, who will need to be attentive to preventing falls (see chapter 15).

Lacerations in association with falls have been shown to be decreased by legislation which provides an incentive to return glass bottles, apparently because there is less broken glass in the environment (Baker et al. 1986). The implication is that keeping a community free from broken glass by any means would reduce injury from falls.

Groups which provide child care for young children (church nurseries, etc.) should not use donated infant furniture if it is in disrepair or no longer has working restraints and should use facilities where other hazards to children have been reduced or eliminated.

10.C.7 Designers, Architects, Builders, and Engineers

Window and screen design should preclude a child's falling through; any opening should be smaller than 4 inches. Gates intended to bar access to stairways should be inexpensive, easy to install and use, and should remain in place with pressure. Consideration might be given to making stair gates a built-in feature of new housing. Gates should not be an injury hazard themselves. For example, wide-V-shaped accordion-style gates, no longer manufactured for sale but still available as used items, permit head entrapment as do gates with vertical slats wider than $2\frac{3}{8}$ inches. Current gate designs have failed to prevent some falls down stairs in infant walkers. Alternatives to the current walker that limit range might be designed. Walkers too wide to go through standard doorways in a home should be less hazardous than many current designs.

Soft surfaces at the bottom of stairs would reduce injury from falls. An energy-absorbing surface at the bottom of the basement stairs could be made a standard architectural feature, for instance. Shrubs or flower beds planted beneath windows provide forgiving surfaces should a child fall.

A lightweight, inexpensive helmet that would be attractive to children and protective during a number of different recreational activities (e.g., bicycling, horseback riding, skateboarding, playing ball) would be a major advantage since the fall injuries of most concern are head injuries (see chapters 6, 11, and 16).

Surfaces that children are likely to fall against contribute to injury. Coffee tables may be involved disproportionately. Appealing furniture might be designed free of sharp angles and edges; the most favorable geometry for roundness of edges still needs to be worked out. Safety glazing should be used for all windows and glass doors accessible to children.

Those designing and building furniture and play equipment for infants and children can make fall injury less likely by reducing heights, by increasing stability, by including easy-to-use and hard-to-remove restraining devices, and by attending to the surfaces underlying the furniture and equipment. Traditional designs for equipment such as changing tables and high chairs must be reevaluated in light of injury hazards. Bunk beds should have guardrails which extend at least 5 inches above the mattress on all four sides and a ladder secured to the frame (CPSC 1987) (see also section 9.C.7).

Bathtubs and shower stalls should be designed with slip-resistant surfaces. At least two grab bars should be securely mounted at different heights beside a bathtub, and one in every shower stall. Accessories such as towel bars and soap dishes should also be securely mounted (CPSC 1979). Tubs and showers should be free of sharp edges; cushioned edges would be an improvement.

Guardrails along open stairways, platforms, porches, walkways, etc., must be constructed with the size and climbing ability of young children in mind. The openings between members must be sufficiently narrow to prevent the body from slipping through as well as to prevent head entrapment. Therefore, the dimensions should be such that a 4-inch sphere will not pass through any opening (Stephenson 1988). The guardrail must also be tall enough so that a child cannot fall over the top. To the same end, guard members should be difficult to climb (e.g., vertical pickets as opposed to horizontal bars). Fixed ladders on farm structures should be out of a young child's reach or fitted with a special barrier to prevent access.

Design standards that might prevent many stair-fall injuries—important for all age-groups but particularly lethal among the elderly—are beginning to receive much-deserved attention. Stairs are safer and falls fewer when the steps are readily seen, the treads are large enough to provide adequate footing, and the handrail is reachable and graspable (Pauls 1984). Handrails designed for toddlers and preschoolers should be 28 to 32 inches high; those for older children and adults can be from 34 to 42 inches high. Handrails should be round and have a diameter from $1\frac{1}{4}$ to 2 inches—at the small end if designed for children. (See figures 10-1 and 10-2). Stairs that meet the needs of adults are important in preventing childhood injury because falling adults might drop infants or fall on children. However, additional work is needed to identify aspects of design needed to meet the peculiar needs of children on stairways, such as lowering freestanding handrail heights to discourage children from swinging on them and falling.

More than half of people treated in emergency rooms for injuries sustained while using bleachers are younger than 15. Typical school bleachers challenge the capabilities of adult users and even more so those of children. Upgrading design standards—for instance, to consider the needs of children in recommending riser height, to decrease the likelihood of falls, to make proper installation and maintenance easy, and to safeguard against collapse—is likely to prevent many future injuries.

10.C.8 Business and Industry

Furniture and play equipment for infants and children should conform to CPSC guidelines and to the most rigorous of voluntary standards. Manufacturers might make safe use a more prominent part of their marketing and labeling strategies. The risk associated with infant walkers appears excessive, and elimination is suggested (Stoffman et al. 1984; Kavanagh and Banco 1982; Birchall and Henderson 1988; Rieder et al. 1986).

Standards for residential facilities, especially single-family homes, have traditionally been less rigorous than for multifamily dwellings and public buildings. Given the large number and high cost of fall injuries occurring at home, it makes sense to invest in designs that will prevent injury. Many such designs, for example, functional handrails along stairways, are not expensive. Support for injury prevention among organizations of home builders would expedite the adoption and dissemination of such changes in the building codes.

10.C.9 Mass Media

An upsurge in toddler falls from windows is a predictable spring event. Timely public-awareness campaigns through print and broadcast media might prompt parents or landlords to provide adequate barriers (e.g., win-

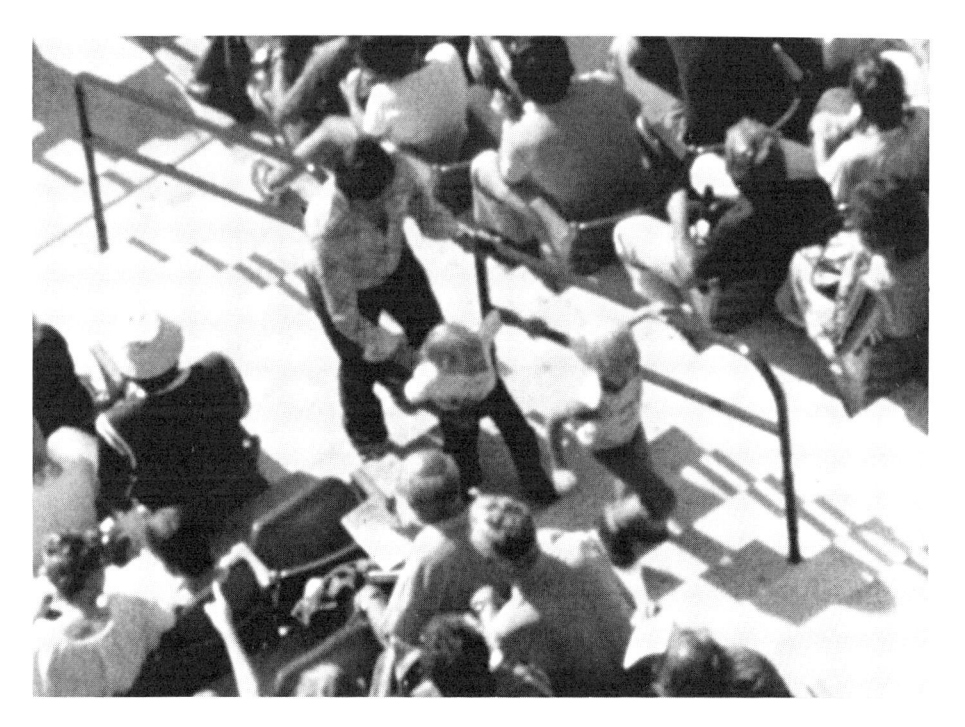

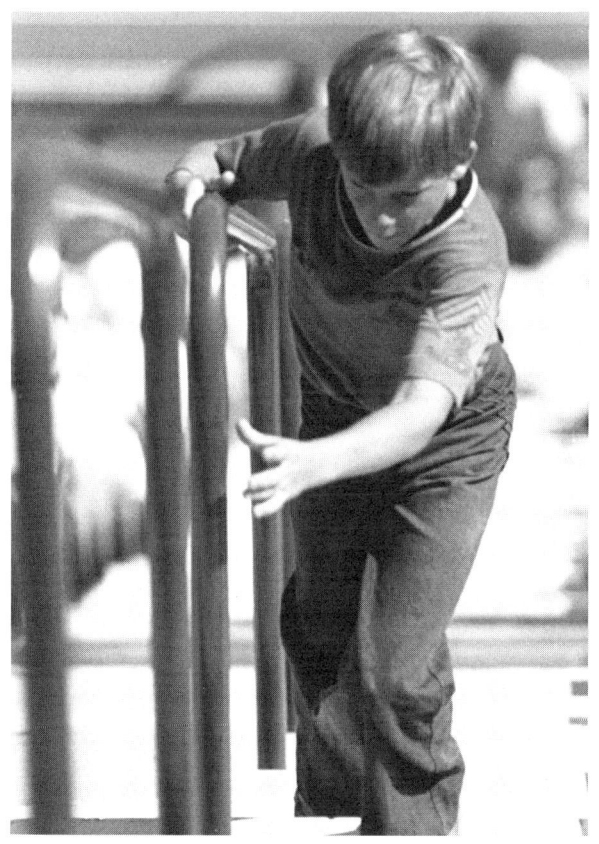

FIGURE 10-1. *The small stature and handgrip of children must be considered when handrails are designed. A frame from the documentary film* The Stair Event *shows handrails installed in a stadium. (From Pauls 1989. Copyright 1989 by J. Pauls. Reprinted by permission.)*

FIGURE 10-2. *A handrail diameter of 1.75⟩ is graspable by a child. (From Pauls 1989. Photo by L. Smith. Copyright 1989 by J. Pauls. Reprinted by permission.)*

dow guards or sturdy screens) across upper-story windows. Similarly, the hazards of infant walkers around stairways and sources of heat and the utility of stairway gates might be highlighted in public-service announcements.

Families with infants who are featured in television programming or other visual media should have fall-prevention devices and practices in place for their role-modeling effect.

References

American Academy of Pediatrics. 1987. *Health in Day Care: A Manual for Health Professionals.* Elk Grove Village: Ill.: American Academy of Pediatrics.
Archea, J, et al. 1979. Guidelines for Stair Safety. *National Bureau of Standards Building Science Series 120.* Washington, D.C.: U.S. Dept. of Commerce.
Association of School Business Officials International. 1986. *School Safety Handbook*, revised version. Reston, Va.: Association of School Business Officials.
Baker, MD, et al. 1986. The impact of "bottle bill" legislation on the incidence of lacerations in childhood. *Am J Public Health* 76(10):1243–1244.
Bergner, L, et al. 1971. Falls from height: A childhood epidemic in an urban area. *Am J Public Health* 61(1):90–96.
Birchall, MA, and Henderson, HP. 1988. Babywalkers and infant burns. *Br Med J* 296(6637):1641.
Canada Mortgage and Housing Corporation. 1981. *Safety in the Home.* Ottawa, Ontario: Canada Mortgage and Housing Corporation.
Child Accident Prevention Foundation of Australia. 1987. *Guidelines on Safety in Family Day Care Homes.* Melbourne, Australia: Child Accident Prevention Foundation of Australia.
Clark, AJ, and Webber, GM. 1982. Accidents involving glass in domestic doors and windows in England and Wales. *Accid Anal Prev* 14(4):293–303.
Consumer Product Safety Commission. 1979. *Bathtub and Shower Injuries.* Product Safety Fact Sheet 3. Washington, D.C.: Consumer Product Safety Commission.
Consumer Product Safety Commission. 1987. *Bunk Beds.* Product Safety Fact Sheet 71. Washington, D.C.: Consumer Product Safety Commission.
Consumer Product Safety Commission. 1988. Hazardous substances and articles; administration and enforcement regulations. 16 *CFR* 1500.18.
Consumer Product Safety Commission. 1989. Warning! Gymnasium bleachers may collapse. *Safety News* December.
Helfer, RE, et al. 1977. Injuries resulting when small children fall out of bed. *Pediatrics* 60(4):533.
James, W. 1988. Despite new regulations, caution a must when baby walkers are used. *Can Med Assoc J* 139(1):73–74.
Joffe, M, and Ludwig, S. 1988. Stairway injuries in children *Pediatrics* 82(3 pt. 2): 457–461.
Kavanagh, CA, and Banco, L. 1982. The infant walker: A previously unrecognized health hazard. *Am J Dis Child* 136:205–206.
Nimityongskul, P, and Anderson, LD. 1987. The likelihood of injuries when children fall out of bed. *J Pediatr Orthop* 7(2):184–186.

Pauls, JL. 1989. Are functional handrails within our reach and grasp? *Southern Building*, September, p. 20.
Pauls, JL. 1984. What can we do to improve stair safety? Part I. *Building Standards* May–June, p. 9.
Ralis, ZA, et al. 1988. Snow-and-ice fracture in the UK, a preventable epidemic, letter. *Lancet* 1(8585):589–590.
Rieder, MJ, et al. 1986. Patterns of walker use and walker injury. *Pediatrics* 78(3): 488–493.
Spiegel, CN, and Lindaman, FC. 1977. Children Can't Fly: A program to prevent childhood morbidity and mortality from window falls. *Am J Public Health* 67(12):1143–1147.
Stephenson, EO. 1988. The silent and inviting trap. *Building Official and Code Administrator*, November/December, pp. 28–33.
Stoffman, JM, et al. 1984. Head injuries related to the use of baby walkers. *Can Med Assoc J* 131(6):573–575.
Williams, AF, and Goins, SE. 1981. Fatal falls and jumps from motor vehicles. *Am J Public Health* 71(3):275–279.
Wissow, LS, and Wilson, MH. 1988. The use of consumer injury registry data to evaluate physical abuse. *Child Abuse Negl* 12:25–31.

Additional Sources of Information

Child Accident Prevention Trust (CAPT)
28 Portland Place
London W1N 4DE
UK
  Fact sheets and reports, including *Child Safety and Housing*, design guidelines for agencies, architects, and builders.

Council of American Building Officials (CABO)
5203 Leesburg Pike
Suite 708
Falls Church, VA 22041
703-931-4533
  Source of information on building codes.

Environmental Design Research Association (EDRA)
733 NE 18th Street
Oklahoma City, OK 73105
405-232-2655
  Annual proceedings contain information on safety in children's environments.

National Institute of Children's Environments (NICE)
23622 Calabasas Road
Suite 149
Calabasas, CA 91302
818-595-7777
  Information for building professionals on home safety.

Network for Injury Prevention in Buildings (NIP)
Box 67, Blue Ridge Hospital
University of Virginia Medical Center
Charlottesville, VA 22901
804-924-5308
  Information on building codes.

11

Animals

11.A Facts

Every year, almost 2% of all children in the United States require emergency room treatment because of an animal bite or sting (Fife et al. 1984). Dog bites are the most common source of injury; researchers in Pennsylvania found that 45% of children surveyed had been bitten by a dog at some time during their life (Beck and Jones 1985). Not all such injuries require hospital treatment, and the majority go unreported to health authorities; even so, there are more than a dozen deaths a year, mostly among young children. Infants younger than 1 year have the highest death rate and typically are attacked by pet dogs in the home. The majority of fatally injured children aged 1 year or older had entered a fenced yard or wandered within reach of a chained dog (Sacks et al. 1989).

Children aged 7-12 are at greatest risk of being bitten by dogs (Beck and Jones 1985), primarily by neighbors' dogs and dogs belonging to their own family. Boys are bitten by neighbors' dogs or strays twice as often as girls, but the sexes have similar rates for bites by their own family dogs. The neck, head, and face, especially the upper lip, are the most common sites of injury. Severe facial injuries occur almost exclusively in children under 10 years old (Karlson 1984).

Male dogs aged 1-4 years have the highest rates of biting; one study estimated that 1 dog in 38 causes an injury resulting in hospital attention (Nixon et al. 1980). Working and sporting dogs (Parrish et al. 1959) and certain breeds of dog are especially likely to bite: German shepherds and collies have especially high rates of biting, and dogs of mixed breeds tend to have lower rates (Hanna and Selby 1981). Recent media and legislative attention has focused on particularly damaging attacks by pit bull terriers (Lockwood 1986). One study of dog bite-related fatalities found that dogs identified as pit bulls were involved in 42% of all U.S. fatalities in which the breed was known—several times more than any other breed (Sacks et al. 1989). Though less often mutilating, cat and rat bites are common, and a variety of other mammals that children come into contact with bite sometimes. Pets that are especially likely to bite children include ferrets, which are often unpredictable and have caused extremely severe facial injury in infants.

Of the diseases associated with animal bites, rabies is the most serious and is found most commonly in bats, raccoons, and skunks. Cats are even more likely than dogs to have rabies, possibly because they are less apt to be vaccinated. Cases of human rabies are now rare, due in part to postexposure treatment given each year to tens of thousands of people bitten by animals that may be rabid. Mammal bites may also result in tetanus or in serious infection with bacteria from the animals' mouths (Jaffe 1983). Other bites that may be serious include snakebites and scorpion stings; the latter can prove fatal to infants. Stings of insects such as bees and wasps can cause life-threatening reactions in anyone allergic to them.

In one study of farm children, 40% of all injuries treated in the hospital were caused by animals (Cogbill et al. 1985). Eye injuries from horned animals often have severe consequences. Medications for animals, even house pets, are not provided in child-resistant containers. They are therefore a potential source of poisoning in young children (see chapter 8).

Horseback riding is an important source of severe and sometimes fatal head injury. Children account for one-fifth of all deaths (probably about 40 per year), with more than 80% of their deaths attributed to head injury (Bixby-Hammett and Brooks 1990). The annual number of horse-related injuries among U.S. children exceeds 10,000, with rates in girls greater than those in boys. Although the upper extremity is the most common site of injury, the majority of hospital admissions involve head injury (Grossman et al. 1978). Defective tack contributes to some falls. The fact that many riders fail to use an adequate helmet is a major contributor to head injury; in addition, the failure to fasten chin straps sometimes causes loss of a helmet. Traditional riding hats are inadequate, but Snell and ASTM have standards for equestrian helmets that set requirements for energy attenuation and retention. The Snell standard, for use in harness racing and other equestrian sports, applies to helmets for adults and youths, not young children. Current helmets that meet the rigorous Snell standard are considered unacceptably heavy by some riders. The ASTM standard aims to ensure adequate head protection with a helmet that is light and comfortable. The U.S. Pony Club requires ASTM-approved helmets for all activities. The American Horse Show Association and several other groups will require junior competitors to wear ASTM-approved helmets starting in 1991. Approved helmets should be worn at all times while riding.

11.B Developmental Considerations

11.B.1, 11.B.2, and 11.B.3 Infants, Toddlers, and Preschoolers

Young children cannot defend themselves against attack by an animal. The incidence of both dog and cat bites that come to medical attention appears to be highest for children under 5 years old (Hanna and Selby 1981). Young children have an increased risk of being bitten on the face, head, or neck, at least partly because of their small size. These bites are especially serious because of their potential to be disfiguring. In addition, some breeds of dogs with large and powerful jaws are able to fracture an infant's skull. Young children are most likely to be bitten by their own family dog in their own home. Although the child is often blamed for the animal's behavior, many bites are unprovoked or occur during forms of play expected at the child's developmental level (Lauer 1982). Dogs are the animal most commonly associated with serious childhood injury, probably because of the number of dog-child contacts, but other animals deserve mention because of the severity of occasional incidents. Toddlers may be kicked or otherwise assaulted by large farm animals (Cogbill et al. 1985). Roosters have caused skull fractures by pecking (Preiser and Lavell 1987), and pet ferrets have attacked and mutilated sleeping infants (Paisley and Lauer 1988). Whether or not cats occasionally inadvertently smother infants by lying on their faces is controversial (Kearney et al. 1982).

11.B.4 and 11.B.5 Elementary School Ages and Young Adolescents

Dogs are favorite animals for many school-age children, and the dog-bite rate remains quite high; one survey found that 20% of children between the ages of 6 and 11 had been bitten in the past year (Beck and Jones 1985). The percentage was even higher among those who owned dogs. Children cannot be relied upon to avoid being bitten, for example by staying away from fenced or chained dogs. Even children in these older age-groups are most often bitten by a neighbor's dog or their own, not by a stray, and boys are more commonly involved than girls. Older children and adolescents who ride horses and children on farms are often granted independence in dealing with large animals. Their size, strength, and judgment are not always equal to the task. More than one-fourth of all horse-related injuries are to persons under the age of 15 (Bixby-Hammett and Brooks 1990), and nearly one in five serious injuries among farm children in one series resulted from a fall from a horse (Cogbill et al. 1985).

11.C Opportunities for Protection

STRATEGIES FOR PREVENTING ANIMAL-RELATED INJURIES
(high-priority strategies are indicated by a △)

Reducing Exposure to Dangerous Animals
- △ Avoid adoption of dog breeds most likely to bite.
- △ Assure that all susceptible pets are vaccinated against rabies.
  Increase licensing fees for dog breeds most likely to bite.
  Encourage families with young children to neuter male dogs or to avoid adopting them.

Provide incentives for neutering animals with dangerous traits.

Do not have ferrets in homes with children.

Maintain physical barriers between young children and large farm animals.

Enforce animal-control laws and laws prohibiting dogfighting.

Increasing Use of Protective Gear

△ Require use of equestrian helmets that meet ASTM or Snell standards.

Other

Teach children not to tease or annoy animals, even family pets, and not to approach fenced or chained dogs.

Package medicine for pets in child-resistant packages.

11.C.1 Schools and Child Care Centers

Animal-safety units can be incorporated into school safety-education programs; these should stress proper behavior with pets and particular local hazards, such as wild animals, rabid animals, poisonous snakes, or sea creatures. Children in rural or farming communities should be taught safe practices to use around farm animals and the importance of wearing adequate helmets when horseback riding. Schools should also establish policies concerning the use of animals in classrooms, dogs and other animals allowed on school grounds, and reporting and first aid procedures for children bitten on school grounds (ASBO 1986).

11.C.2 Health Care Providers

Health care providers should be prepared to advise parents about which pets are safest for families with young children (e.g., avoid ferrets, some breeds of dogs) and that children should be taught to avoid unsupervised animal contact. Even family dogs with no biting history should be closely attended around very young children. Children should be taught to crawl to safety when large animals attack (Busch et al. 1986).

Pediatricians and other health care providers should advise the use of a riding helmet with strap fastened during horseback riding for those patients who ride, identify individuals who should not ride competitively due to medical conditions, and develop and disseminate criteria for allowing resumption of riding after an injury (Brooks and Bixby-Hammett 1988). Emergency medical personnel and physicians treating children who struck their heads falling from a horse should be cognizant of the possibility of cervical spine injury. Thoracolumbar spinal injuries also occur when riders fall on their buttocks.

11.C.3 Public Agencies

Agencies should conduct surveillance studies to determine the prevalence of rabies and of animal bites (wild and domestic) in their area. Areas with new or ongoing problems should consider establishing a bureau of animal control or similar department if not already established, or designating animal control as a priority if a suitable center of activity already exists. Rat-control initiatives must be included in many urban areas where young children are bitten by rats. Agencies in areas with animal-control problems should establish enforcement units or assign responsibility for enforcing agency policy among existing personnel. State and local licensing, vaccination, bite-reporting, leash-law, and sanitation requirements should be included in enforcement efforts (Berzon 1978).

Agencies responsible for animal control in areas where rabid animals are found should educate the public as to the risk of exposure to wild animals, the need to keep domestic animals' rabies immunizations current, and the importance of obtaining medical attention if bitten by a wild animal (CDC 1982) or a domestic animal that might be rabid. Offering pet owners immunization clinics is likely to increase the rate of immunization among domestic animals. Sites harboring animals known to be rabid, such as skunks, foxes, and bats, should be cleaned out, and steps should be taken to prevent reinhabitation (AAP 1987).

Leash laws and stray animal control, helpful in reducing the number of potentially aggressive or rabid animals in a community, may help reduce the problem of animal bites as well. Many children are bitten in and around their homes, however, and thus may not be affected by such laws (Karlson 1984). Animal shelters and kennels should encourage neutering; incentives may be helpful. Persons adopting reproductively intact young male dogs should be advised that these dogs pose the greatest hazard of aggressiveness (AAP 1987), and that this risk can be reduced by neutering.

Stringent licensing requirements and high fees applied to dog breeds identified as biters (through surveillance data or other sources) may reduce the dog population likely to cause injury (Karlson 1984). Increased fees and penalties and licensing prerequisites such as rabies vaccination, which increase the cost of owning a pet, may be effective in reducing the number of pet owners not committed to responsible ownership (Berzon 1978).

Agencies involved with horseback riding programs or horse shows should require adequate helmets for all riders. Agencies involved with farm animals should teach animal safety or coordinate farm safety-education programs with local schools.

11.C.4 Legislators and Regulators

Communities should have comprehensive animal-control ordinances which establish licensing and vaccination requirements and clarify other issues of pet and wild animal control (e.g., leash laws, sanitation requirements, definition of public nuisance) (Berzon 1978). Strong enforcement of existing laws, such as leash laws, and greater efforts to stop dogfighting, such as making it a felony in all states, may help to decrease attacks by dogs.

Sale and ownership of pets deemed to be excessively hazardous should be prohibited. One such example is ferrets, which exhibit unpredictable behavior, including attacking sleeping children; may form feral populations destructive to local animals; and for which no proven rabies vaccine exists (Paisley and Lauer 1988). Vicious-dog laws have been enacted by several states and localities following dog attacks on children and adults. Their impact should be monitored, and, if favorable, similar laws should be adopted in other jurisdictions.

Veterinary medicines should be included in the Poison Prevention Packaging Act; child-resistant caps should be required on all veterinary medicines and hazardous products (Glickman et al. 1982) (see chapter 8).

11.C.5 Law Enforcement Professionals

Law enforcement officers often assist other delegated authorities in dealing with animal control and in enforcing state and local regulations. Where no separate authority exists, police should take responsibility for animal-control enforcement and regulation. This may include issuing dog and cat licenses.

Law enforcement professionals may also be involved in investigating dogfights. Although not intended to affect children directly, dogfighting provides an incentive for breeding and training dogs to be vicious. It should be discouraged.

11.C.6 Voluntary Organizations

Groups sponsoring horseback riding should require approved protective headgear and adequate supervision. Other safe riding practices include regular inspections of tack; proper fit of tack on the horse; proper boots (with a heel); and proper fit of the stirrup to the boot so that the foot neither sticks in the stirrup, precluding emergency dismounting, nor slips through the stirrup, causing the fallen rider to be dragged.

Youth groups can teach large-animal safety to farm children and responsible pet ownership to all. Organizations like the Humane Society promote responsible animal ownership and help with animal control by caring for strays.

11.C.7 Designers, Architects, Builders, and Engineers

Head injuries suffered in falls from horses are an important cause of serious recreational injury. Riding helmets have now been developed in both hunt-style and jockey-style designs to meet ASTM's 1988 standard, and at least one manufacturer is said to be working on western-style protective headgear. New designs that make helmets even more acceptable to riders are welcome, as are designs that offer more protection, for instance to the lower back part of the skull (Brooks and Bixby-Hammett 1988). Derby hats and top hats, used in dressage activities, are still not generally available as helmets meeting the ASTM standard. Although such hats are rarely worn by children, adult riders are powerful role models. Designers should develop protective helmets in these styles if possible, or such styles should be replaced by a protective helmet in another style.

Release catches have been designed for English saddles to prevent riders from dragging if caught in the stirrups. These do not work for children, however, who may be too light to open the release in a fall, nor for most riders, who do not ride in English saddles (Bixby-Hammett and Brooks 1990). Research could be useful in designing release catches for children's saddles. Breakaway stirrups and body protectors are other devices mentioned for preventing injuries to riders. Their use for children could be evaluated.

Buildings that house animals should have proper flooring (impervious material, roughened to prevent slips, constructed to allow drainage); proper fencing and gates (strong and durable); solid-walled alley and loading chutes; and even and diffused lighting to keep animals from being skittish (Farm Safety Association 1985).

11.C.8 Business and Industry

Breeders and pet shops should be encouraged to emphasize dog breeds not likely to bite. Owners who buy dogs of a breed known to bite should be informed that a chain may not be an adequate restraint—a securely enclosed and locked pen that children can't enter is preferred (Sacks et al. 1989). Pet shop owners can stop carrying breeds of dogs or other animals known to attack humans, such as ferrets.

Riding establishments that cater to child riders should have appropriate tack and supervisory personnel and should insist that riders wear approved protective headgear. They should be prepared to deal appropriately with medical emergencies resulting from a kick, fall, or trampling.

11.C.9 Mass Media

A bitten child must often face rabies shots. The message that pets should be immunized against rabies needs to be repeated over and over again.

The loving interdependence of children and pets often portrayed on the printed page and the screen needs to be balanced with facts about animal-induced injuries and about animals and breeds most likely to injure. Nonsensational media coverage of vicious dog attacks may help reduce the macho image of some dogs and thereby reduce demand.

Media portrayal of modern horseback riders wearing protective headgear—including cowboys, cowgirls, and rodeo riders—could do much to make helmets acceptable.

References

American Academy of Pediatrics. 1987. *Injury Control for Children and Youth*. Elk Grove Village, Ill.: American Academy of Pediatrics.
Association of School Business Officials International. 1986. *School Safety Handbook*, revised version. Reston, Va.: Association of School Business Officials.
Barber, HM. 1973. Horse-play: Survey of accidents with horses. *Br Med J* 3:532-534.
Beck, AM, and Jones, BA. 1985. Unreported dog bites in children. *Public Health Rep* 100(3):315-321.
Berzon, DR. 1978. The animal bite epidemic in Baltimore, Maryland: Review and update. *Am J Public Health* 68(6):593-595.
Bixby-Hammett, DM, and Brooks, WH. 1990. Common injuries in horseback riding: A review. *Sports Med* 9(1):36-47.
Brooks, WH, and Bixby-Hammett, DM. 1988. Prevention of neurologic injuries in equestrian sports. *Physician and Sportsmedicine* 16(11):84.
Busch, HM Jr, et al. 1986. Blunt bovine and equine trauma. *J Trauma* 26(6):559-560.
Centers for Disease Control. 1982. Rabies—Mid-Atlantic States. *MMWR* 31(44):592.
Cogbill, TH, et al. 1985. Farm accidents in children. *Pediatrics* 76(4):562-566.
Farm Safety Association. 1985. *Safety with Farm Animals*. Fact Sheet No. F-008. Guelph, Ontario: Farm Safety Association.
Fife, D, et al. 1984. Northeastern Ohio Trauma Study: II. Injury rates by age, sex, and cause. *Am J Public Health* 74(5):473-478.
Glickman, NW, et al. 1982. Accidental poisoning of children by veterinary drugs. *Natl Clgh Poison Control Cent Bull* 26(2):1-2.
Grossman, JA, et al. 1978. Equestrian injuries: Results of a prospective study. *JAMA* 240(17):1881-1882.
Hanna, TL, and Selby, LA. 1981. Characteristics of the human and pet populations in animal bite incidents recorded at two Air Force bases. *Public Health Rep* 96(6):580-584.
Jaffe, AC. 1983. Animal bites. *Pediatr Clin North Am* 30(2):405-413.
Karlson, TA. 1984. The incidence of facial injuries from dog bites. *JAMA* 251(24):3265-3267.
Kearney, MS, et al. 1982. Can a cat smother and kill a baby? *Br Med J* 285:777.
Lauer, EA, et al. 1982. Dog bites: A neglected problem in accident prevention. *Am J Dis Child* 136:202-204.
Lockwood, R. 1986. Vicious dogs: Communities, humane societies, and owners struggle with a growing problem. *Humane Society News* Winter.
Nixon, J, et al. 1980. Dog bite injuries to children: Potential rabies threat to Australia. *Med J Aust* 1(4):175-176.
Paisley, JW, and Lauer, BA. 1988. Severe facial injuries to infants due to unprovoked attacks by pet ferrets. *JAMA* 259(13):2005-2006.
Parrish, HM, et al. 1959. Epidemiology of dog bites. *Public Health Rep* 74:891.

Preiser, G, and Lavell, TE. 1987. Rooster attacks on children. *Pediatrics* 79(3): 426–427.

Sacks, JJ, et al. 1989. Dog bite-related fatalities from 1979 through 1988. *JAMA* 262(11):1489–1492.

Additional Sources of Information

ASTM (formerly known as the American Society for Testing and Materials)
1916 Race Street
Philadelphia, PA 19103
215-299-5400
Equestrian helmet standard.

Farm Safety Association
340 Woodlawn Road
Suite 22
Guelph, Ontario N1H 7K6
Canada
519-823-5600
Information on farm and animal safety.

Farm Safety for Just Kids
716 Main Street
PO Box 458
Earlham, IA 50072
515-758-2827
Information on farm and animal safety.

Humane Society of the U.S.
2100 L Street, NW
Washington, DC 20037
202-452-1100
Guidelines on animal-control ordinances, training for enforcing dogfight-prohibition laws.

The Institute of Agricultural Medicine and Occupational Health
The University of Iowa
Iowa City, IA 52242
319-335-4415
Information on farm and animal safety.

Snell Memorial Foundation
PO Box 493
St. James, NY 11780
516-862-6545
Equestrian helmet standard.

U.S. Pony Clubs, Inc.
893 Matlack Street
Suite 110
West Chester, PA 19382
215-436-0300
Information on equestrian safety and injury data.

12

Firearms

12.A Facts

Childhood shootings from both powder and nonpowder firearms (those using gas, air, or a spring to propel ammunition, including BB guns) constitute a major public health problem. As with firearm injuries in the overall population, childhood shootings have usually been discussed in a fractionated fashion; that is, homicides, suicides, and unintentional shootings have been separated from each other. This disaggregation has masked the severity of the firearm problem as a major killer of children. The 658 gun-related deaths of U.S. children under age 15 in 1986 represented almost 7% of all childhood injury deaths and were exceeded only by deaths from motor vehicles, drowning, and house fires.

In 1986, 40% of children's firearm deaths were homicides (see table 12-1), accounting for one-quarter of all child homicides. The likelihood that child homicide will be accomplished with a firearm increases with age, from 3% of homicides for children younger than 1 to 62% for children 10 to 14 years old.

The suicide rate among the young has been rising dramatically for the past few decades. Most of the increase among adolescents and young adults is accounted for by the increasing rate of suicide with guns (Boyd and Moscicki 1986). Guns are used in 56% of child suicides overall, and the percentage increases in older victims (see chapter 14).

Firearms are the third leading cause of unintentional injury deaths in the 10- to 14-year age-group, exceeded only by motor vehicles and drowning. Firearms cause one-sixth of all unintentional injury deaths in this age-group. The fatality rate for males is seven times the rate for females. The death rate from unintentional shootings is higher for males aged 13-17 than for males at any other age.

The apparent intent of the shooter in firearm deaths varies with the age of the victim (see table 12-1). At ages 0-4 the majority of firearm fatalities are homicides. At ages 5-9 the majority of firearm deaths are unintentional. At ages 10-14 gun deaths are almost evenly divided among suicides, homicides, and unintentional shootings.

Many of the unintentional shootings of children occur when the injured child or another child is playing with a loaded gun found in the home

Table 12-1. Firearms as Source of Childhood Injury Mortality, by Age, in U.S., 1986

	\< 1	1–4	5–9	10–14	Total 0–14
Intent					
Unintentional	3	31	57	143	234
Intentional					
Homicide	8	51	53	152	264
Suicide	0	0	1	142	143
Unknown	0	0	0	17	17
Total firearm deaths	11	82	111	454	658
Percentage of injury deaths caused by firearms	0.9	2.4	5.2	16.3	6.8

Number of Deaths, by Age

Source: National Center for Health Statistics, 1988.

(Wintemute et al. 1987; Keck et al. 1988). Sometimes the gun is mistaken for a toy. Guns that are left loaded and unlocked in a home, kept there for purposes of protecting the family, too often result in family tragedies instead of family security (Heins et al. 1974; Christoffel and Christoffel 1986).

Nonpowder firearms cause at least 14,000 injuries annually among children younger than 15, with boys accounting for four out of five of the injuries. In fact, nonpowder guns cause three times as many injuries to children as powder guns. Although nonpowder-firearm injuries generally are less severe than those from powder guns, fatalities and permanent disabilities do result. These guns are often purchased as toys and are not regulated at the federal level and only loosely by local jurisdictions (Christoffel et al. 1984).

Firearm injuries associated with hunting appear to affect the young disproportionately. As many as one-quarter of hunting firearm injuries are fatal. If North Carolina is typical, one in seven shooters in hunting fatalities is a male younger than 15 (Cole and Patetta 1988). Although many young shooters and wounded hunters lack formal gun-safety training, fluorescent clothing, or adult supervision, it is unclear how many injuries these measures would prevent. Fatalities occur in the presence of all three and among very experienced hunters (Heins et al. 1974).

Strategies to prevent firearm injuries and deaths include restricting the manufacture and sale of certain types of guns, mandating a waiting period and thorough background check before a gun can be purchased, designing guns so children can't pull the trigger, and providing safety locks and a mechanism to indicate that the gun is loaded. Nonpowder firearms could be regulated and/or banned from children's use, and toy guns should be easily discernible from real guns.

12.B Developmental Considerations

12.B.1 Infants

Infants do not operate guns themselves but are victims of gun violence. About 3% of all infant homicides are committed with a firearm.

12.B.2 and 12.B.3 Toddlers and Preschoolers

Toddlers and preschoolers are fully capable of operating many firearms. They can never be expected to identify guns as dangerous or to resist the temptation to play with them. Many guns, especially handguns, have no safety locks, and the trigger pulls are often so light that toddlers and preschoolers can fire them. Most of the unintentional gun deaths among children of this age are self-inflicted. The marketing of small, concealable handguns to women (see section 12.C.8) may increase children's access to guns and is even more hazardous if these models do not have built-in safety locks.

12.B.4 Elementary School Ages

School-age children are well able to find guns that are kept at home to "protect" the household but remain unlikely to avoid them or to handle them safely. Gun play with realistic toy guns is common, particularly among boys. This play may be transferred to the use of real guns when they are available, often with the child failing to understand that the gun is not a toy or that the gun is loaded. Nonpowder guns also become favored "toys" among older boys, so a high number of injuries from these weapons might be expected, given current gun designs and foreseeable misuse by children.

12.B.5 Young Adolescents

The gun homicide rate begins to climb, particularly for males, as children enter adolescence. In some areas, guns are purchased by young males for self-protection and/or crime and may even be taken to school. Suicide with guns also increases, and unintentional gun deaths reach their highest rates in the adolescent male population. Using guns may be one way adolescent males seek to assume adult roles.

12.C Opportunities for Protection

> STRATEGIES FOR PREVENTING FIREARM INJURIES
> (high-priority strategies are indicated by a △)
>
> *Reducing the Number of Guns in the General Environment*
> △ Pass federal and state laws restricting the manufacture and sale of certain guns that have low legitimate utility and high injury rates.

Pass a federal law requiring a thorough investigation and waiting period before a gun can be purchased.

Increase enforcement of laws restricting the purchase of guns by specified persons.

Place restrictions on the sale of nonpowder guns for use by children.

Sustain the ban on the manufacture and sale of plastic handguns and other new technologies that can elude metal detectors.

Altering the Gun Itself

△ Require that guns be child-resistant, to lower the likelihood that a young child could discharge a gun.

Require guns to have safety locks.

Require design that indicates whether guns are loaded.

Personalize guns with a device that allows only owners to fire them.

Make toy guns easily identifiable.

Educating Gun Owners

△ Educate potential buyers of handguns that the danger of shooting someone in the family usually exceeds the value of the gun in protecting against an intruder.

Educate current gun owners and potential buyers of the need to store guns unloaded and locked.

12.C.1 Schools and Child Care Centers

Child care should never be provided in the homes of individuals who keep a loaded gun for protection. Current data suggest that the risk of a child finding a loaded gun and discharging it far outweighs whatever protective benefit might be provided (Morrow and Hudson 1986; Rushforth et al. 1975; Kellermann and Reay 1986; Keck et al. 1988).

Schools should be aware of the risks that guns pose to their students. There are reported incidents involving even grade schools, and certainly middle or junior high schools, in which children brought guns to schools. Some schools have instituted policies preventing students from wearing coats or carrying book bags while inside the school, on the theory that weapons can easily be concealed in these items. Other schools, in cities with high rates of gun violence among schoolchildren, use metal detectors to keep guns out. Curricula that teach nonviolent conflict-resolution skills are being tested and may help to reduce firearm injuries.

Schools should carefully examine any curriculum offered to them on gun safety. Some of these curricula have been prepared by progun organizations, ostensibly for the purpose of safety training, but they may also have the effect of introducing children to the concept of personal possession of firearms and acclimatizing children to the alleged benefits of possessing guns.

Schools have the opportunity to educate children in the legal facts about the possession of guns. Much misinformation exists about the meaning of the Second Amendment to the U.S. Constitution and about other gun laws. Providing valid information, such as the fact that the Second Amendment does not give each citizen the right to possess whatever gun he or she chooses (as is often misstated by progun organizations), can help lead to rational and safe gun policies in the future. (For further reading on the Second Amendment issue, see *Quilici et al. v Village of Morton Grove*, listed in the additional sources of information).

Schools should encourage the formation of student organizations, similar to Students Against Drunk Driving, that demand a gun-free environment. For students living in cities, their risk of death may be greater from firearms than from drunk drivers.

12.C.2 Health Care Providers

Guns in the home are a serious health hazard (Keck et al. 1988). Many families with children keep guns. In a survey conducted in one pediatric clinic, 38% of families reported having at least one gun in their home (Patterson and Smith 1987). It is alarming to note that half the guns were kept loaded, and some families freely admitted the gun was accessible to children.

Physicians and others who care for children have an opportunity and a responsibility to inform the parents of their patients about the dangers of keeping a loaded gun in the home. Although most children's physicians are not firearm experts, they are experts in child health hazards and in child development. Acquisition of a gun should be discouraged. For those families who continue to keep a weapon in the home, there should be clear instructions that the gun should always be kept unloaded, separated from the ammunition, and locked away. Older children may use a gun to commit suicide. Health care providers should be alert to any signs of depression a child exhibits (see section 14.C.2) and work with parents and child to keep guns inaccessible.

Male children have a particularly high rate of injury from nonpowder firearms (Christoffel et al. 1984), and parents of boys should be advised that even nonpowder guns are hazardous.

In addition to counseling parents, health care providers should work to educate society in general, and lawmakers in particular, that guns represent a substantial public health problem and the gun issue should be dealt with as such.

12.C.3 Public Agencies

Guns are a major health hazard, and in some population groups are the leading cause of death. Health departments should therefore recognize firearm issues as being within their jurisdiction. The vital statistics section of the health department, particularly at the state level and in urban areas, should aggregate gun mortality data from all causes (i.e., homicide, suicide, unintentional, and undetermined) and report the aggregated data to the public and to decision makers to emphasize that firearms are a legitimate public health issue.

Health agencies and state legislatures should consider making firearm injuries reportable to health departments. Currently, in some areas, these injuries must be reported by health care providers to the police but not to health authorities. Reporting to health departments would facilitate epidemiologic studies on gun-related morbidity and the cost of such injuries.

State agencies responsible for licensing persons to own and carry guns should investigate applicants to the fullest extent specified by law. This often requires cooperation from and coordination of a number of agencies and data systems; an efficient system should be in place. Once a gun is placed in the hands of a person, efforts to regulate its use can have little effect.

Community-based programs to prevent violence, offered by health departments or other municipal agencies to children at high risk, may help to prevent firearm injuries.

12.C.4 Legislators and Regulators

Perhaps the clearest opportunities for reducing the number of childhood shooting injuries reside within the authority of legislators and regulators. Lawmakers should focus on limiting the manufacture and sale of guns rather than allowing guns to be sold indiscriminately and then trying to regulate their use. Assault weapons should be banned. A federal law requiring a 7-day waiting period before a gun sale and a thorough background check on the purchaser should be passed without delay.

State and federal laws can and should be enacted that limit the availability of guns in general, thereby limiting their availability to children as well. As a positive example, plastic handguns that look and feel like toys and do not trigger metal detectors were banned before they had the chance to permeate the market. It is foreseeable that such guns would have been mistaken for toys by children, and that their proliferation would result in increased childhood gun deaths. Certain widely available guns have low legitimate utility and high risk for causing injury, such as the Saturday night special—by definition an inexpensive, inaccurate, short-barreled, low-caliber handgun that has often been used in crimes. States should consider enacting laws similar to one enacted in Maryland in 1988 (Teret et al. 1990), which provides that the only handguns that may be manufactured or sold in the state are those listed on a roster developed by a nine-person board appointed by the governor. The intent of the law is to prohibit the manufacture or sale of Saturday night specials.

States should allow localities that perceive they have a gun problem to legislate tighter restrictions on the availability of guns locally. States with preemptive laws prohibiting such home rule should repeal those laws.

Guns are now regulated at the federal level by the Bureau of Alcohol,

Tobacco, and Firearms within the Treasury Department. The bureau must exercise greater care to ensure that those licensed to sell firearms are not permitting illegal sales (e.g., to minors).

Neither the Consumer Product Safety Commission nor any other agency charged with protecting the health and safety of the public has jurisdiction over firearms. This results in a lack of regulatory power to reduce the injury toll caused by guns. Jurisdiction should be given to and regulations should be promulgated by an agency that will examine product alterations such as required safety latches, trigger locks, and load indicators.

The availability of nonpowder guns as toys for children can be regulated locally or federally. Local jurisdictions can ban the sale of nonpowder firearms for use by children. The Consumer Product Safety Commission, which currently has the authority to regulate these products but has decided not to do so in the past (Christoffel and Christoffel 1989), should be urged again to do so.

12.C.5 Law Enforcement Professionals

Law enforcement personnel have a great deal of credibility with regard to guns. They have influenced legislation and other policy in the past and should continue to do so. In this context, law enforcement officers might support legal restrictions on the private ownership of certain types of guns, particularly nonsporting firearms. Such restrictions might include banning the manufacture, sale, and possession of assault weapons and poorly detectable handguns; restrictions on sales, thorough background checks, and waiting periods prior to purchase; limitations on where a firearm can be carried and by whom; registration or reporting of all firearm purchases; confiscation power for the police under certain circumstances; and the repeal of preemptive laws that prevent localities from enacting firearms legislation more restrictive than existing state legislation. While these measures do not address firearm injuries to children exclusively, one of the benefits of decreasing the number of firearms in children's environments will certainly be a reduction in the number of such injuries.

Many firearm laws are already in place. Enforcement should be given high priority. In areas where background checks are required before purchase, the responsibility is often assigned to law enforcement agencies. A system for accomplishing thorough checks while preserving the citizen's rights is a necessity. Current data systems are often inadequate or poorly accessible, limiting the utility of the law.

Law enforcement personnel have mistakenly shot children carrying toy guns which they supposed to be real. Support for making toy guns unmistakable is logical (see section 12.C.8).

Police are frequently summoned to scenes of domestic violence. Children may become the unintended victims, often after a series of altercations, when adults threaten each other with guns (Nelson 1984). Police might be trained to recognize the potential for child maltreatment when investigating family fights and to initiate intervention by child-protective services when indicated.

Law enforcement professionals have ready access to children through school and community programs. They are in an ideal position to raise community awareness about handgun hazards, to discourage the acquisition of firearms for "protection," to assist schools in prohibiting guns on school property, to advise families who choose to own guns about proper handling and storage, and to provide private citizens with a safe way to dispose of firearms.

Law enforcement agencies often have valuable data on firearms and the harm they inflict. Such data could be analyzed and presented to the community and to lawmakers.

Finally, many law enforcement officers carry firearms home. Their handling and storage practices must be impeccable to protect both their own children and visitors.

12.C.6 Voluntary Organizations

Gun-safety courses have been touted as an approach to decreasing injury risks associated with recreational uses of guns. Certainly, those who choose to use guns should know how to use them with the least possible risk to human life. However, it is unlikely that even the highest-quality training can eliminate the risk for children associated with handling guns. Some shooters in hunting accidents, for instance, have had gun-safety training (Cole and Patetta 1988). Even police officers, who are trained gun users, and their family members have been injured (Heins et al. 1974), and unintended shootings have occurred in police stations (Morrow and Hudson 1986). Further, gun-safety courses for children are likely to increase their interest in obtaining and using guns. By way of analogy, high school driver education actually increases motor vehicle deaths by putting more young drivers on the road (Robertson and Zador 1978). Organizations should avoid offering programs that attract children to guns. Children cannot consistently use guns safely.

All groups offering programs for children should explicitly prohibit the carrying of guns by adult leaders or participating children. Involvement in a community group may promote positive attitudes and steer children away from violence and firearms. Some organizations target violence-prevention or youth-development programs to high-risk youth. Such programs should be used and evaluated for effectiveness (National Committee for Injury Prevention and Control 1989).

12.C.7 Designers, Architects, Builders, and Engineers

A number of design innovations have been suggested to make guns more difficult to fire unintentionally. These include changing the trigger so that small children cannot exert enough pressure to fire the gun, adding or changing locking or safety mechanisms so they must be subverted deliberately in order to fire, personalizing the gun by a device that allows firing only by the owner, and modifying the gun's design so that even school-age children can tell when it is loaded.

12.C.8 Business and Industry

Marketing tactics suggesting that women need to purchase guns to assure their personal safety will, if successful, increase firearm injuries to children, since guns kept by women who have or take care of children may be accessible to those children. Given the lack of evidence that keeping a handgun does decrease a woman's risk of injury, such marketing should be stopped. Stores that sell guns might provide the customer with verbal and written instructions about safe handling and storage practices and advise customers to choose guns with safety locks and to purchase lockable storage devices.

Toy guns that can be mistaken for real guns put children at substantial risk (see figure 12-1). Children carrying facsimiles may mistakenly be assumed to be armed and therefore may be shot by others. Children may

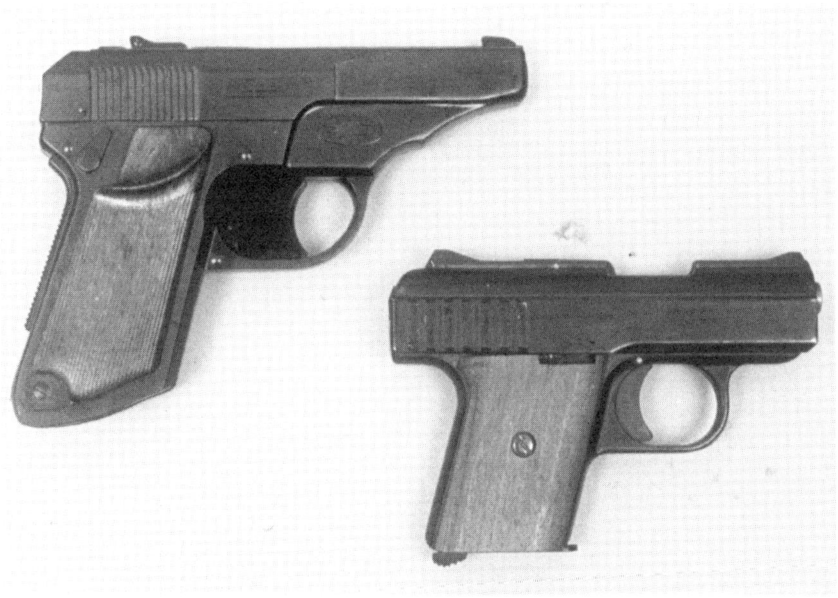

FIGURE 12-1. *One of these firearms is a real gun, confiscated by the police after being used in a residential shooting; the other is a toy. They are difficult to distinguish, even for an adult. (Photo by G. Wintemute. Reprinted by permission.)*

mistake a real gun for a toy and shoot themselves or others. Since children easily imagine in their games that even a stick is a gun, there is no reason to believe they would not accept toy guns that were clearly identified as toys. Toy gun manufacturers and Congress have embarked on a plan to identify toy guns visually by means of an orange plug in the barrel (U.S. Congress 1988). Though laudable because of the concern it shows for preventing childhood injury, this standard is likely to be inadequate because of several shortcomings—for instance, the orange plug may be invisible from the side or from a distance. The toy gun in figure 12-1 has a barrel marking that complies with the 1988 regulation; it cannot be seen from this angle. Even more creative leadership is needed in this area.

Some toy stores have chosen not to offer realistic toy weapons, even when they are available. The public is likely to support such efforts when the reasons are made clear. Nonpowder firearms marketed as toys carry a high risk of injury; businesses can choose not to offer them.

12.C.9 Mass Media

No other childhood injury issue generates more intensely emotional debate and polarized pressure than firearms. Members of the media can make an important contribution by getting the message out that guns kill not only adults but also children. This may be particularly needful in small, non-urban markets where media representatives and their audiences may not be as conscious of the issue as in large urban areas. In addition, the media can stress that firearms are a public health as well as a criminal justice problem.

Television and film scripts might be carefully scrutinized for behaviors that model facile or casual handling or use of firearms (e.g., guns "hidden" under pillows, or games of Russian roulette). These behaviors and other deliberate or subtle messages that promote gun use to children might be avoided. Advertisements in children's magazines admonishing children to use guns safely should be considered in this category unless it can be clearly shown that the benefits outweigh the risks.

References

Boyd, JH, and Moscicki, EK. 1986. Firearms and youth suicide. *Am J Public Health* 76(10): 1240–1242.

Christoffel, KK, et al. 1984. Childhood injuries caused by nonpowder firearms. *Am J Dis Child* 138:557–561.

Christoffel, KK, and Christoffel, T. 1986. Handguns: Risks versus benefits. *Pediatrics* 77(5):781–782.

Christoffel, T, and Christoffel, KK. 1989. The Consumer Product Safety Commission's opposition to consumer product safety: Lessons for public health advocates. *Am J Public Health* 79(3):336–339.

Cole, TB, and Patetta, MJ. 1988. Hunting firearm injuries, North Carolina. *Am J Public Health* 78(12):1585-1586.

Heins, M, et al. 1974. Gunshot wounds in children. *Am J Public Health* 64(4):326-330.

Keck, NJ, et al. 1988. Characteristics of fatal gunshot wounds in the home in Oklahoma: 1982-1983. *Am J Dis Child* 142(6):623.

Kellermann, AL, and Reay, DT. 1986. Protection or peril? An analysis of firearm-related deaths in the home. *N Engl J Med* 314:1557-1560.

Morrow, PL, and Hudson, P. 1986. Accidental firearm fatalities in North Carolina, 1976-80. *Am J Public Health* 76(9):1120-1123.

National Center for Health Statistics. 1988. *Vital Statistics of the United States, 1986.* Vol. 2, Mortality, pt A. Dept. of Health and Human Services Publication No. (PHS) 88-1122. Washington, D.C.: U.S. Government Printing Office.

National Committee for Injury Prevention and Control. 1989. *Injury Prevention: Meeting the Challenge.* New York: Oxford University Press.

Nelson, KG. 1984. The innocent bystander: The child as unintended victim of domestic violence involving deadly weapons. *Pediatrics* 73(2):251-252.

Patterson, PJ, and Smith, LR. 1987. Firearms in the home and child safety. *Am J Dis Child* 141(2):221-223.

Robertson, LS, and Zador, PI. 1978. Driver education and fatal crash involvement of teenaged drivers. *Am J Public Health* 68:959.

Rushforth, NB, et al. 1975. Accidental firearm fatalities in a metropolitan county (1958-1973). *Am J Epidemiol* 100(6):499-505.

Teret, SP, et al. 1990. The passage of Maryland's gun law: Data and advocacy for injury prevention. *J Public Health Policy* 11(1):26-38.

U.S. Congress. 1988. Federal Energy Management Improvement Act. Public Law 100-615, Section 4, Penalties for entering into commerce of imitation firearms.

Wintemute, GJ, et al. 1987. When children shoot children: 88 Unintended deaths in California. *JAMA* 257(22):3107-3109.

Additional Sources of Information

Quilici et al. v Village of Morton Grove, 695 F. 2d 261 (7th cir. 1982). Concerns the Second Amendment.

Center to Prevent Handgun Violence
1225 Eye Street, NW
Suite 1100
Washington, DC 20005
202-289-7319
 Information on handgun safety, childhood injuries, suicide, gun control, and guns and the Constitution. Also school curriculum, community programs, and media packages.

Centers for Disease Control
Division of Injury Epidemiology and Control
Center for Environmental Health and Injury Control
Atlanta, GA 30333
404-488-4646
 Information on intentional and unintentional firearm injuries.

Educational Fund to End Handgun Violence
Box 72
1100 Maryland Avenue, NE
Washington, DC 20002
202-544-7227
Information on children and handguns.

International Association of Chiefs of Police
1110 North Glebe Road
Suite 200
Arlington, VA 22201
Information on firearms for law enforcement professionals.

National Criminal Justice Reference Service
National Institute of Justice
Rockville, MD 20850
800-851-3420 or 301-251-5500 (in Maryland)
Information on school violence, gun control, police firearms training, and working with victims.

National School Safety Center
16830 Ventura Boulevard
Suite 200
Encino, CA 91436
818-377-6200
Information on weapons in schools.

National Society to Prevent Blindness
500 East Remington Road
Schaumburg, IL 60173
800-221-3004
Information on nonpowder firearm injuries.

13

Assaults

13.A Facts

Most assaults on children are perpetrated not by strangers but by parents or others responsible for their care. Such assaults are but one manifestation of a more pervasive problem of child maltreatment usually referred to as child abuse. Though difficult to define precisely, child abuse reflects a social judgment that a particular way of treating a child is inappropriate by community standards and puts the child in jeopardy of serious harm (Garbarino et al. 1986a). In addition to overt assault with an intent to harm, child abuse includes physical punishment which goes beyond the community's standards; sexual molestation; psychological maltreatment in the form of verbal assault, rejection, terrorizing, missocializing, and emotional neglect; and the failure to meet basic needs. The criterion for labeling a pattern of behavior as child abuse is not that it results in injury but rather that a reasonable adult would know that it probably will result in injury.

This chapter focuses on physical assaults that create a high risk of injury and thus excludes neglect as well as sexual exploitation and psychological maltreatment that can lead directly to developmental "injury" and indirectly to injuries sustained because of related emotional and psychological problems. Other types of assault are discussed in the relevant chapters—for instance, inflicted burns are discussed with other burns in chapter 7, intentional poisoning with other poisonings in chapter 8, and firearm injuries in chapter 12.

Most parents assault their children. They do so in the name of "discipline" or "punishment." At least three-quarters of parents have used some form of violence on their children. In a 1975 survey, 20% of parents admitted they had hit their child with an object; 4% had "beaten up" a child; and 3% had used a gun or knife to threaten or injure their child (Gelles and Straus 1988). Through much of history, assaults by parents against children were considered acceptable or even desirable unless they produced severe injuries. Even then, injury or death might have been treated as "accidental" because it was inflicted in the course of "appropriate discipline." Community standards have changed. Assault with intent to cause injury and assault which is likely to produce injury are no longer considered acceptable. Public and private child welfare and health agencies are called upon to identify and prevent inappropriate assault, or child abuse.

Child abuse is an inconsistently recognized, incompletely reported, and variously defined cause of injury that is poorly quantified by analyses of standard health statistics. Special studies are required to count even recognized and reported child assaults, and even these almost certainly underestimate the problem significantly. Using a parsimonious definition (i.e., cases of demonstrable harm recognized by professionals), the National Incidence Study published by the National Center on Child Abuse and Neglect (NCCAN) found more than 300,000 cases of injury resulting from physical abuse of children younger than 18 in 1986, an increase over identically defined data collected in 1980, which may be accounted for by increased recognition (NCCAN 1988). Stated another way, at least 1 child in 200 suffered physical injury, sometimes resulting in death or permanent impairment, from assault by a parent or other adult caretaker during the year. The incidence of recognized abuse-related injury increases with the child's age, with the highest rates among preadolescents and adolescents; however, the fatality rate from abuse or neglect is highest for children younger than 3 years of age.

When an assault results in death, it is classed as homicide, a category that includes child abuse as well as death from injuries inflicted by people who are not responsible for a child's care—a sibling, for example, or an arsonist. In 1986 there were more than 600 homicides involving children under 5 years of age, the majority of which probably would be considered the result of child abuse or neglect. Analyses of U.S. mortality data for the years 1980 through 1985 reveal that homicide is the leading cause of injury death for infants and accounts for 10% of all injury-related deaths for children younger than 15 years of age (Waller et al. 1989). It is clear that assaults against children and youth by parents and other caregivers are a significant feature of the injury problem.

Assault-related injuries are most often recognized in multiproblem, high-stress families with low income, few resources, and difficulty relating to others and the outside world. However, child abuse is very prevalent and is by no means limited to that setting.

13.B Developmental Considerations
13.B.1 Infants

Infants are "perfect victims" in the sense that they are defenseless and unable to communicate. Of course, they are also perfect victims in the sense that they elicit sympathy and are not blamed for being assaulted as older children often are. Even adults who justify assault as a form of discipline for older children may consider it inappropriate for infants.

While infants are less likely than older children to be physically assaulted, they account disproportionately for fatalities—with a death rate nine times the rate for 3- to 5-year-olds (NCCAN 1988). Infants are vulnerable to particularly damaging types of injury, such as brain damage resulting from shaking (Caffey 1974). What is more, the private nature of most infant care creates opportunities to obscure the source and cause of injury. A number of assault deaths are probably not recognized and are consequently mislabeled (Bass et al. 1986).

Caring for an infant is very demanding, particularly for the parent with few resources faced with a fussy or colicky baby. This inherent difficulty interacts with belief in the use of assault to discipline children. No form of "punishment" is developmentally appropriate for infants. One study found that a group of high-risk young mothers spanked their 6-month-olds approximately once per week (Olds et al. 1986). Researchers have identified spanking at 6 months of age as a risk factor predictive of subsequent child abuse.

13.B.2 and 13.B.3 Toddlers and Preschoolers

The use of assault as a form of discipline becomes commonplace among parents by the toddler period and continues throughout childhood. The socialization issues of toilet training, eating, obedience, and household maintenance drive much of the day-to-day interaction of parents with their young children. As children acquire the skills of walking and talking, they become more independent and less certainly controlled by their parents. Spanking and slapping become routine. Surveys of parents suggest that well over 80% of 3- and 4-year-olds experience physical force as an aspect of parenting (Straus et al. 1981). In a cultural climate in which physical assault is condoned as a form of discipline, conditions of high stress and low resources may produce assault-related injuries.

Mothers are somewhat more likely than fathers to assault their children, and boys are more likely to be assaulted than girls (Straus et al. 1981). Of special concern is the finding that young children who live with a nonbiologically related adult (stepparent or other substitute parent) are at greater risk of abuse than children living with both natural parents. Some researchers speculate that this results from a "sociobiological" predisposition for people to provide better care for children in whom they have a genetic investment (Daly and Wilson 1985).

13.B.4 Elementary School Ages

As children reach elementary school age, socialized behavior appears, and adults gradually switch to reasoning and social punishments for discipline (e.g., withdrawal of privileges, confinement to a room). Violence as a form of discipline decreases modestly, but it is still used with four out of five children. According to the National Incidence Study, however, the rate of physical abuse continues to rise—perhaps because children become more powerful (and thus require more physical force to subdue), and their plight is more likely to be known outside the family (because of attendance at school) (NCCAN 1988). While fatalities decrease markedly, in part reflecting the fact that the older child's body tolerates more physical punishment than the infant's, moderate injuries increase.

13.B.5 Young Adolescents

"Only" about one-half of young adolescents are struck by a parent, and fatalities are rare; however, the rate of recognized injury is higher than at earlier ages. Most observers now believe that the dynamics of adolescence create the need for the family to renegotiate roles and rules. The result is that some families formerly stabilized begin to deteriorate, and a new wave of assault may occur (Garbarino et al. 1986b). A small but measurable percentage of parents report that they have "beaten up" a child, sometimes repeatedly, and some admit they have used a gun or knife to threaten their child (Straus 1975). The enlarging social sphere and extreme dependence on same-sex peer groups of young adolescents also put them at risk, especially the boys, for assault by peers. Fights are a common interaction. When knives or especially guns are available, the fights may be lethal.

13.C Opportunities for Protection

> STRATEGIES FOR PREVENTING ASSAULTS
> (high-priority strategies are indicated by a △).
>
> *Changing Adult Behavior*
> △ Teach parents and other caregivers nonassaultive means of disciplining children.
> △ Provide home health visitors and/or other support systems to high-risk families.
>
> *Changing the Social Environment*
> Pass and enforce legislation prohibiting corporal punishment in schools.
> Require careful screening of child care personnel and foster and adoptive parents.
> Develop a coordinated network of agencies promoting prevention programs.
>
> *Identifying At-Risk Children*
> △ Train professionals who deal with children to recognize signs of assault and to report suspected assaults immediately.

13.C.1 Schools and Child Care Centers

Preventing child abuse in the professionally run child care setting depends upon three things: staff screening (cooks, janitors, and other support personnel who have access to the children should be included), set standards of care, and good supervision. Screening can be accomplished by interviewing, observing on-site, checking references, and posing hypothetical situations as a way of identifying high-risk individuals.

To prevent abuse, the child care center or school should have strong norms about discipline (no hitting, no belittling, no locking children in rooms, no tolerance of peer assault, etc.). Corporal punishment should be prohibited. Without clear and firm standards of care, the social environment can deteriorate, and adults slide toward abuse and neglect. Training might be provided to help teachers and staff members learn alternate, nonviolent disciplinary techniques.

The professional is responsible for supervising nonprofessional staff, monitoring peers and administrative superiors, and ensuring that the social environment is well managed. A professional must take the time to observe other staff with children unannounced. Parents must have free access to children. Staff must be able to observe each other and share responsibility. Child maltreatment thrives in conditions of isolation and secrecy. If allegations of abuse are made, the staff should cooperate fully with the investigators. Of course, the better the child care center's policies, operating practices, screening, and records, the easier this will be. Good rapport with parents also makes a difference. Any allegation of abuse can set off parent panic and community hysteria, so effective communication is critical, as is firm but gentle treatment of an accused staff member. Legal counsel is very important. One way to prepare for the eventuality of a child abuse allegation is to become part of an active professional network or association so that material and moral support are forthcoming in a time of crisis.

Child care workers and teachers, as well as all other professionals who deal with children, must be alert for signs of abuse — too many bruises too often, bruises not in the places expected after a simple fall, bruises shaped like objects, burns, depression, changes in performance or behavior. In all jurisdictions, professionals who report suspected abuse in good faith are protected from civil action for doing so, and in most states they are required to report. Early reporting is a crucial preventive measure because most deaths follow repeated assaults.

Schools and child care centers can teach nonviolent problem-solving methods or conflict-resolution techniques in an effort to help students develop alternate ways of dealing with each other and with their own children in the future.

13.C.2 Health Care Providers

Health professionals have a special responsibility to diagnose maltreatment and nonfatal assault before it becomes fatal or permanently damaging. When it comes to identifying child abuse, the most important theme is "eyes, ears, and minds open" to the reality of child maltreatment. Children suffering from abuse or neglect at home may exhibit clear signs: bruises, burns, injuries which don't fit the offered explanation, bizarre behaviors, or a sense of self or reality that reflects parental definitions or attitudes that are abusive, as in "I'm a bad bad girl and I don't deserve to get any lunch. My dad told me so." Beyond these clear warning signals, the health professional must be alert to the ebb and flow of each child's life as evident in how that child acts with peers and adults, what the child says about himself or herself, and what parents say and do to and about the child. Particularly important to recognize is the close linkage between the abuse of women (spouse abuse) and child abuse. Whenever one is detected, the other should be suspected and close inquiry made.

Home health visitors may help to prevent assaults (Olds et al. 1986). They visit the family early in the child's life on a regular basis, have a "normal" (rather than problem) focus, and can use their relationship with the family to intervene effectively and unobtrusively. All health care providers involved with children should know and be able to teach nonassaultive discipline techniques (Christophersen 1980).

13.C.3 Public Agencies

On an individual level, if professionals dealing with children suspect that a child is being abused, they should discuss their suspicions with their supervisor (if they have one) and/or share their concerns with a colleague. Sharing the decision-making responsibility is an important safeguard for the individual professional and for the child and his or her family. The responsible professional must then decide if the suspicions are plausible. If so, institutional support must be sought. Every state authorizes a particular public agency, usually the official child protective-service agency, to receive and investigate reports. Many states provide a toll-free hotline for reporting child abuse. Getting action on behalf of a child may require persistence. If a case of suspected child abuse is not verified at the time of the initial report, the professional who reported should continue to monitor the child, if possible. An initially unverifiable situation may become clearer as evidence mounts or conditions in the child's life deteriorate. Many cases found to be unsubstantiated are substantiated within three years following subsequent reports.

Many systems are terribly overburdened, particularly in large cities. One consequence is a deterioration in the speed, depth, and perhaps even accuracy of investigations. This can be very frustrating for the person reporting a case of suspected child abuse. Services may be completely inaccessible to rural families (Daro 1988). In addition, the resource crunch facing many public protective agencies calls out for everyone who cares for children to join the battle for improved funding and administration. Building the capacity of protective services and other human-service agencies is a high priority for advocacy.

The National Committee for Prevention of Child Abuse (NCPCA) has developed a national agenda for preventing child abuse, available in a booklet from the NCPCA (see additional sources of information). The recommended package includes support services and education for all new parents (ideally beginning prenatally), personal safety instruction for all schoolchildren, treatment for child victims, public awareness of child abuse, expanded professional understanding of the causes and consequences of abuse, and the development of a coordinated network of agencies promoting prevention programs. With a chapter in all 50 states, the NCPCA is a valuable resource for agencies hoping to develop programs to prevent child abuse. Additional programs that are likely to complement or enhance basic child abuse prevention efforts include those designed to prevent domestic violence, to provide shelters and other alternatives for battered women and their children, to provide parenting programs and parent support services to families at high risk for violence, to prevent and treat substance abuse, and, more generally, to prevent poverty.

13.C.4 Legislators and Regulators

Legislation is important in setting standards for care and providing the resources necessary to promote attainment of those standards by parents. It also is a means of ensuring that foster and adoptive parents are carefully screened to avoid abuse and neglect.

Legislation that clearly prohibits the use of physical force as a disciplinary method in schools should be passed in every state. About half the states have accomplished this goal. Problems with children are not solved by having their teachers strike them. The state, and its education system, which for long periods of a child's day acts in a parental role, should assure that it is a model parent. Beyond this, states should move toward a total ban on assault against children—by anyone. In this, the lead of Sweden and Austria might be followed; these countries have enacted such bans as part of educational campaigns.

13.C.5 Law Enforcement Professionals

Law enforcement personnel provide an important entry point into the prevention-oriented systems. They can be trained to be alert to risk factors for children that are uncovered in the course of responding to other issues, such as spousal violence or negligence-related injuries. Law enforcement officers can work to establish a climate of trust and cooperation with children as well as with other professionals and the community.

In jurisdictions where law enforcement agencies have the primary role in initial investigation of alleged child abuse, the officers involved should be given specific training. Some police departments are issuing teddy bears to their personnel for use during child-abuse cases. These stuffed animals seem to make children more secure during times of crisis and increase communication between the police and children.

13.C.6 Voluntary Organizations

Voluntary organizations can sponsor prevention programs that focus on substituting nonassaultive modes of conflict resolution and discipline for the use of force. The National Committee for Prevention of Child Abuse (see additional sources of information) is a primary source and rallying point for such efforts.

Self-help groups with professional backup such as Parents Anonymous have demonstrated their ability to help some parents decrease the frequency of abusive behavior while increasing their feelings of self-esteem and knowledge of child behavior. Parent aide programs also appear to have a positive effect on parents' confidence, social contacts, attachment, and disciplining expectations and behaviors (Meyers and Bernier 1987). Both can be important parts of a comprehensive approach to prevention.

13.C.7 Designers, Architects, Builders, and Engineers

An extensive role in preventing assaults to children for those who design products and environments has yet to be defined. Certainly, modifications which prevent hot-water heaters or taps from discharging dangerously hot water would prevent deliberate hot tap-water burns (see chapter 7), and modifications of firearms might prevent some intentional as well as unintentional shootings (see chapter 12).

It is possible that products and environments that reduce the difficulty of child care may decrease parental stress and reduce the likelihood of child battering. The infant swing is often recommended for quieting a colicky baby, for instance. Carrying a baby in a soft infant carrier attached to the parent's body has been shown to reduce total crying time (Hunziker and Barr 1986). Such design alternatives may be useful but have not been directly evaluated as interventions to prevent child abuse.

13.C.8 Business and Industry

Employees can be offered a number of services which are likely to reduce family violence of all kinds. Such services include drug- and alcohol-abuse detection, treatment, and rehabilitation; parenting programs; spouse-abuse prevention; and courses in conflict resolution.

Making it easier for employees to obtain reasonable child care is likely to reduce parental stress and decrease tensions which lead to assaults on children. Other family-oriented workplace policies, such as flexible work schedules, generous benefit packages, and parental leave, can help parents deal with dual roles and should decrease family dysfunction and violence (Meyers and Bernier 1987) as well as enhance productivity.

13.C.9 Mass Media

The mass media play an important role in defining what is normal for parents and children. Conducting a media campaign to highlight the problem of assault and the availability of intervention services is one thing that television, radio, and print media can do. An additional approach is to monitor the content of entertainment programs to ensure that they set models for behavior and offer suggestions for alternatives to assault in family relationships.

References

Bass M, et al. 1986. Death-scene investigation in sudden infant death. *N Engl J Med* 315(2):100–105.
Chaffey, J. 1974. The whiplash shaken infant syndrome: Manual shaking by the extremities with whiplash-induced intracranial and intraocular bleedings, linked with residual permanent brain damage and mental retardation. *Pediatrics* 54:396–403.
Christophersen, ER. 1980. The pediatrician and parental discipline. *Pediatrics* 66(4):641–642.
Daly, M, and Wilson, M. 1985. Child abuse and other risks of not living with both parents. *Ethology and Sociobiology* 6:197–210.
Daro, D. 1988. *Confronting Child Abuse*. New York: The Free Press.
Garbarino, J, et al. 1986a. *The Psychologically Battered Child*. San Francisco: Jossey-Bass.
Garbarino, J, et al. 1986b. *Troubled Youth, Troubled Families*. New York: Aldine.
Gelles, RJ, and Straus, MA. 1988. *Intimate Violence: The Causes and Consequences of Abuse in the American Family*. New York: Simon and Schuster.
Hunziker, UA, and Barr, RG. 1986. Increased carrying reduces infant crying: A randomized controlled trial. *Pediatrics* 77(5):641–648.
Meyers, M, and Bernier, J. 1987. *Preventing Child Abuse: A Resource for Policymakers and Advocates*. Boston: Massachusetts Committee for Children and Youth.
National Center on Child Abuse and Neglect. 1988. *Study Findings: Study of National Incidence and Prevalence of Child Abuse and Neglect: 1988*. Washington, D.C.: National Center on Child Abuse and Neglect.
Olds, D, et al. 1986. Preventing child abuse and neglect: A trial of nurse home visitation. *Pediatrics* 78(1):65–78.
Straus, MA, et al. 1981. *Behind Closed Doors: Violence in the American Family*. Newbury Park, Calif.: Sage.
Waller, AE, et al. 1989. Childhood injury deaths: National analysis and geographic variations. *Am J Public Health* 79(3):310–315.

Additional Sources of Information

Ciccheti, D. 1989. *Child Maltreatment: Theory and Research on the Causes and Consequences of Child Abuse and Neglect*. New York: Cambridge University Press.
Finkelhor, D, et al. 1983. *The Dark Side of Families*. Beverly Hills: Sage.

Finkelhor, D., et al. 1986. *A Sourcebook on Child Sexual Abuse.* Newbury Park, Calif.: Sage.

Garbarino, J, and Gilliam, G. 1980. *Understanding Abusive Families.* Lexington, Mass.: Lexington Books.

Kempe, CH, and Helfer, RE (eds.). 1987. *The Battered Child.* Chicago: University of Chicago Press.

Orbach, I. 1988. *Children Who Don't Want to Live.* San Francisco: Jossey-Bass.

Wissow, LS. 1990. *Child Advocacy for the Clinician: An Approach to Child Abuse and Neglect.* Baltimore: Williams and Wilkins.

American Association for Protecting Children (AAPC)
Children's Division of the American Humane Association
PO Box 1266
Denver, CO 80201
303-695-0811 or 800-2-ASK-AHA
  Resources include data and materials on program and policy development.

American Bar Association (ABA)
Center on Children and the Law
1800 M Street, NW
Washington, DC 20036
202-331-2250
  Information on legal and judicial issues relating to child abuse and neglect, including child fatality review committees.

Kempe National Center for the Prevention and Treatment of Child Abuse and Neglect
1205 Oneida Street
Denver, CO 80220
303-321-3963
  Resources include training and consultation services.

National Center on Child Abuse and Neglect (NCCAN)
Clearinghouse on Child Abuse and Neglect Information
PO Box 1182
Washington, DC 20013
202-245-0586 or 703-821-2086 (clearinghouse)
  Resources include data, reviews of research, evaluation studies of programs, guides for law enforcement professionals and other professionals.

National Committee for Prevention of Child Abuse (NCPCA)
332 South Michigan Avenue
Suite 1250
Chicago, IL 60604
312-663-3520
  Resources include information on self-help groups, disabled children and child abuse, and strengthening families through the workplace.

National Conference of State Legislatures
1050 17th Street
Suite 2100
Denver, CO 80265
303-623-7800
  Resources include annual summary of state legislation pertaining to children, youth, and families; topics include child abuse and neglect, domestic violence, suicide.

National Criminal Justice Reference Service
National Institute of Justice
Box 6000
Rockville, MD 20850
800-851-3240 or 301-251-5500 (in Maryland)
  Information for law enforcement professionals and others on child abuse, sexual abuse, domestic violence.

National Woman Abuse Prevention Project
2000 P Street, NW
Suite 508
Washington, DC 20036
202-857-0216
  Educational and training materials on child maltreatment and woman abuse.

Parents Anonymous
National Office
6733 South Sepulveda
Suite 270
Los Angeles, CA 90045
800-421-0353
   Self-help groups for caregivers.

14

Suicide and Suicide Attempts

14.A Facts

Of all causes of childhood death, suicide may well be the most tragic because, in addition to the loss of life, it often reflects a prior period of hopelessness and personal problems. Suicide in children under 15 years of age is much less common than in older adolescents, and therefore has been the subject of less research. Yet the suicide rate in the 10- to 14-year age-group has increased dramatically in recent years, more than doubling between 1980 and 1985.

In the 10- to 14-year age-group, suicide is now the sixth leading cause of death in males; in 1986 there were 197 suicides in males and 54 in females. The rate in whites in this age-group is about twice that in blacks; Native Americans have the highest rate, more than double the rate in whites. The number of suicides in Native Americans aged 10–14 is exceeded only by deaths related to motor vehicles and drowning. Suicide is rare in children less than 10 years old, but about five deaths annually are so categorized. The spectrum of intent in child suicide, as in older age-groups, ranges from not caring whether one lives or dies to self-destructive thoughts and behaviors to acts calculated to be irrevocable and lethal.

Among males aged 10–14 in the United States, two-thirds of suicides involve the use of firearms and almost one-third are by hanging. Among females, half involve firearms, with hanging and poisoning accounting for about 30 and 15%, respectively. Hanging is the predominant means among Native American children.

Nonfatal suicide attempts are common in teenagers; two surveys found that almost two-thirds of high school students had thought about committing suicide and 8 to 9% had attempted it at some time in their lives (Smith and Crawford 1986; Harkavy Friedman et al. 1987). Such acts typically involve overdoses of medications, notably analgesics and psychotropic agents. Based on hospital admission rates, self-poisoning rates in females begin to rise steeply at about age 12 and reach a peak at age 15 or 16; for males both the rise and the peak occur about three years later. The rates for females are about 50% higher than for males (Trinkoff and Baker 1986).

A history of a suicide attempt or threat is probably the most important predictor of subsequent attempts. Among other important predictors of suicide are depression or manic-depressive illness, abusive use of alcohol or drugs, physical or sexual abuse, hopelessness, impulsivity, and runaway behavior. Precipitating factors in many suicides include disrupted relationships, interpersonal conflicts, crises, losses, and other stresses (Brent 1989). The following list (adapted from Ross and Lee [n.d.] and Brent [1989]) presents common warning signs and high-risk situations leading to suicide:

- Suicide threats
- Statements revealing a desire to die
- Previous suicide attempts
- Sudden changes in behavior (withdrawal, apathy, moodiness)
- Depression (crying, sleeplessness, loss of appetite, hopelessness)
- Final arrangements (such as giving away personal possessions)
- Family disintegration (e.g., loss of parent, abandonment)
- Psychological, physical, or sexual abuse at home
- Substance abuse
- Psychiatric disease
- Suicidal role modeling — suicide by a family member or peer or media portrayal (e.g., television or popular film presenting suicide)

Alcohol intoxication has increased in importance and is now involved in about half of teen suicides (Brent et al. 1987). The availability of a gun in the home is a major determinant of whether a suicide attempt becomes a fatality (Brent et al. 1988).

14.B Developmental Considerations

Children may display suicidal behavior of a number of types: thoughts of suicide, threats of suicide or suicide "gestures," suicide attempts, accomplished suicide, or self-destructive intent disguised as "accidental" injury (Otto 1972). Experts do not agree on how these categories are related. Some believe that without successful intervention, gestures may lead to the accomplished act, while others see these groupings as manifestations of more or less distinct patterns. Important for those interested in injury prevention is the fact that all may lead to injury or death. An act intended as a gesture to mobilize personal support may prove fatal if the child misperceives the lethality of the method or others do not respond in the predicted way.

Explanations for suicide may be grounded theoretically in psychological, biological, or social-environmental theory (Shaw et al. 1987). Whatever the conceptual framework, the suicide of a child or young adolescent represents a failure of normal developmental processes. Children who seek death often come from multiproblem families that appear to be disintegrating, where children feel rejected, and in which communication patterns are seriously distorted (Orbach 1988). Though fleeting suicidal thoughts in childhood are so common as to be considered normal, suicidal plans and acts are not, and a child experiencing such a degree of hopelessness is asking for and in immediate need of supportive intervention.

14.B.1 and 14.B.2 Infants and Toddlers

The first few years of healthy psychological development are dominated by attachment to parent(s) and then garnering the ability to endure brief separation without unbearable insecurity. Quite early, children learn that appearing and disappearing can manipulate the feelings and actions of others. If a secure relationship never develops, or if the child experiences loss of a key figure, the child may be isolated from the start, bereft of the requisite sense of self and self-esteem for normal individuation. A pattern may be set which will later evolve into hopelessness, and the child's anger and aggressiveness may be turned on himself or herself. Also in this very early period a pattern of neglect or abuse by the parent may begin. Children who consider or attempt suicide are much more likely than their peers to report having been abused or neglected (Hibbard et al. 1988).

14.B.3 Preschoolers

Quite early on, children begin to think of death, but at first may misunderstand its meaning. Euphemisms of adults ("He passed away" or "He's sleeping") and the ephemeral nature of life and death on television probably do little to clarify children's understanding. Thought processes at this age are characterized by "magical thinking" in which death is reversible. Young children often wish such a death on those closest to them, who therefore are most likely to thwart their strong desires, and they begin to contemplate and fear their own death—often personified by the many imaginary monsters which may enter the bedroom at night. Preschoolers are capable of suicidal behavior (Rosenthal and Rosenthal 1984), but it is thought to be rare. Some observers who have worked closely with suicidal children believe such behavior is much more common in young children than previously acknowledged. It must not be ruled out, even for preschool children.

14.B.4 Elementary School Ages

During the early school years (ages 5 through 8), the concept of death is a piece of very active psychological work for the child (Otto 1972). Similarly, fleeting thoughts about suicide appear to be common. In one study (Lourie 1967), slightly more than half of a group of children without recognized emotional problems said they had at least once thought about killing themselves. The proportion was even higher among those with recognized emotional problems. Yet suicide remains unusual, or at least rarely recognized, before age 10.

Depression occurs during childhood much more commonly than is noticed by parents, teachers, and other adults, including health care providers. As research proceeds on childhood depression, the more it appears to resemble the syndrome as it occurs in adolescents and adults. Depressed children and adolescents are a high-risk group for suicide. Signs of depression include sleeping or eating problems, apparent lack of energy or interest in school or friends, general deterioration of performance and behavior, complaints of boredom or loneliness, feelings of guilt and expressions of sadness, hopelessness, and emptiness (Shaw et al. 1987). Valid instruments for screening for and diagnosing depression in childhood are available for use by professionals (see 14.C.2). Children with psychiatric disorders or with a family history of psychiatric disturbance, alcoholism, or suicidal behavior are also in high-risk groups.

14.B.5 Young Adolescents

Suicide attempts and suicides become much more common after age 12. This may represent a developmental stage in which the ability to plan and carry out self-killing is added to the wish to do so. Interaction with a psychotic parent or imitation of a suicidal parent or role model may help to trigger the act. Precipitating crises come from the fabric of adolescent developmental tasks — disciplinary actions, family conflicts, school or work problems, estrangement from special friends. These overwhelm the young person whose fundamental needs for security, contact, and love (Otto 1972) have not been met or are too great to be met. The negative aspects of early experience may in some instances prove virtually insurmountable.

The middle-school child, aged 10–13, is at a crossroads. Problems of substance abuse, sexual experimentation, and social adjustment emerge — all of which may lead to guilt, anger, aggression, hopelessness, and suicide. The period of early adolescence may be a last-chance opportunity for those who wish to intervene.

14.C Opportunities for Protection

STRATEGIES FOR PREVENTING SUICIDES
(high-priority strategies are indicated by a △)

Reducing the Availability of Lethal Agents
△ Reduce sales and ownership of firearms.
   Do not keep guns in the home.
   Provide only nonlethal quantities of highly toxic medications to adolescents with emotional problems.

Choose the least toxic drug for treatment of children and adolescents at risk for suicide.

Identifying At-Risk Children

△ Improve recognition of symptoms or characteristics that suggest high risk (e.g., hopelessness, depression, family disruption).

Teach families, school personnel, and health care workers to recognize the circumstances that increase risk (e.g., physical abuse or personal crises).

Treating At-Risk Children

Give special attention to children who have attempted suicide (e.g., admit to hospital rather than discharge from emergency room, develop signed "no-suicide" agreements).

Provide child, adolescent, and family therapy to assist with the "insolvable problem" (Orbach 1986) (e.g., assist in mourning loss or in dealing with child abuse and neglect).

14.C.1 Schools and Child Care Centers

School personnel should be trained to recognize the warning signs of suicide (some of which are listed in section 14.A) and certain events which might precipitate suicidal behavior, as discussed in section 14.C.2. Students who continually go to the school nurse may be calling for attention and should be considered for suicide risk (Otto 1972).

Teachers and support personnel must know how to respond to students who talk about suicide or exhibit suicidal or self-destructive behavior. The best things to do are (1) discuss the suicidal statements or behavior openly and honestly; (2) show interest and support; and (3) get professional help—either persuade the student to get help directly or consult with a professional on how to handle the situation (Ross and Lee n.d.). Schools should have a clearly defined procedure for quick access to psychological or psychiatric consultation in such cases. Materials are available to help school personnel and students deal with suicidal feelings, suicide threats, and suicides; these might be distributed and discussed at separate workshops. Mental health or other agency personnel might present or train teachers to present suicide-intervention programs, as described in section 14.C.3. Active participation of parents should be encouraged (Nelson 1987). School curricula are available to help students develop problem-solving and coping skills.

School personnel should cooperate with other members of the community to develop a community plan to prevent and contain suicide clusters— that is, "a group of suicides or suicide attempts, or both, that occur closer together in time and space than would normally be expected in a given community" (CDC 1988). Many aspects of the plan, discussed in detail in section 14.C.3, would be helpful to follow in the event of a single suicide, as well. The following suggestions are made for school personnel:

1. School officials might announce the deaths of students in an appropriate manner—briefing first the teachers and support staff, then students particularly close to the suicide victims, then the student body, preferably in small groups (e.g., homeroom classes).
2. Teachers, counselors, and students might help identify other students at high risk.
3. Teachers might work with local mental health agencies to get training and support to deal with the suicides and to counsel students as necessary.
4. Hot lines and walk-in counseling centers might be established temporarily at schools or using school personnel.
5. Funeral services should not disrupt the regular school schedule unnecessarily; memorials to the suicide victims installed on school grounds are potentially dangerous as they may unintentionally glorify the decedents' acts.

14.C.2 Health Care Providers

Health professionals have a unique responsibility in suicide prevention. Primary prevention requires promoting healthy relationships between the infant or growing child and the parent(s), in which love, security, self-esteem, and communication flourish. Health professionals have frequent and predictable interactions with families with young children. They have opportunities to detect rejection and to enhance bonding through, for example, assuring early infant-parent contact through "rooming in" on the maternity ward and liberal visiting policies on other hospital wards. They also have the opportunity to identify relationships which are in jeopardy and refer for more intense parenting support.

Secondly, physicians must recognize circumstances which carry an increased risk of suicide (depression, history of neglect or abuse, early loss of a parent, psychiatric condition in the child or family, alcohol or other drug abuse, vague somatic complaints, low self-esteem) (see section 14.A) and ask about suicidal ideation, plans, and past attempts. Questions may be asked directly and simply (Brent 1989). There is no evidence that such questioning is suggestive or itself a precipitating event. On the other hand, there *is* evidence that children and adolescents will reliably answer such questions asked privately by a person with whom they have some rapport (Shaw et al. 1987). When answers to questions about suicidal intent suggest risk, mental health intervention for the child and family is urgent.

Physicians must be particularly sensitive to the signs and symptoms of childhood depression (see section 14.B), make the diagnosis, and provide or arrange therapy. Reliable diagnostic tools are available (e.g., the Children's Depression Inventory [CDI] and the Childhood Depression Scale [CDS]). If a child shows depressive symptomatology on such an instrument when administered twice (Shaw et al. 1987) or if there is a high degree of clinical suspicion, the child should be referred for a structured interview by a clinical psychologist or child psychiatrist using the Children's Depression Rating Scale (CDRS) or the Schedule for Affective Disorders and Schizophrenia for School Age Children. When depression is diagnosed, specific therapy must be initiated. The efficacy of antidepressant drugs in childhood depression is not as clear as it is in adolescence or adulthood, and the use of such drugs, if prescribed, must be supervised by the parent to prevent intentional overdose. Individual, and often family, counseling is a must with or without medication.

Many young persons who commit suicide have been seen by a health professional within a short time of the event (Hawton 1982). It therefore behooves the health professional not only to be aware of high-risk situations and to diagnose and treat childhood depression but also to be sensitive to a history of recent events which might precipitate self-destructive behavior. These include disciplinary or romantic crises and conflicts with parents or at school or work (Shaw et al. 1987). Similarly, prodromal signs (increased tension, restlessness, irritability, oversensitivity, truancy, general deterioration of social behavior [Shaw et al. 1987]) should be recognized for what they may portend while there is time to intervene. If a child leaves notes documenting suicidal intention, gives away possessions, or appears to be making other arrangements for death, these should be taken as urgent signs.

In such a case or following a suicide attempt, an assessment must be made of risk for further suicidal behavior. Risk-rescue tables have been developed for this purpose (Weisman and Worden 1972). Seriousness of intent may be related to risk of repetition and has been found to be greater when plans were made to preclude discovery, extensive preparations were made, and no attempt was made to summon help after the act (Beck et al. 1974). In cases which indicate serious intent, where the patient is upset at having failed, or family members do not respond immediately in a caring way, the patient should be hospitalized until the life situation can be changed and therapy begun even if the injury caused by the suicide attempt is trivial and does not require further medical treatment. When the patient is not hospitalized, a signed "no-suicide" agreement may be helpful to cover the period until the mental health specialist takes over care. The risk of repetition is highest in the first two years following an attempt, and the risk of completion is real. An ongoing treatment plan is essential. Physicians probably misdiagnose many suicidal injuries in children and young adolescents as "accidental" because they do not think children will commit suicide at such an early age. Failure to recognize an injury as intentionally self-inflicted precludes the most appropriate and specific intervention which may prevent further injury.

Physicians put the weapon in the hands of many suicidal persons by the liberal prescription of narcotic and psychotropic drugs. Toxicity of overdose should be considered when drugs are selected and amounts specified. Just as the families of depressed and suicidal young people should be counseled to remove weapons such as guns from the home, so should they remove unnecessary medications. Likewise, suicidal patients should not be given access to means to complete a suicidal act. Window and screen designs should prevent jumping; curtain, closet, and shower rods should break away with weight; and cords, sharp objects, and medications should be inaccessible.

14.C.3 Public Agencies

State and local agencies, such as education, public health, and mental health, can be effective by cooperating with other resources in the community to develop a plan for the prevention and containment of suicide clusters (see section 14.C.1). Guidelines available from the Centers for Disease Control might also be helpful in organizing a community's resources to prevent or respond to a single suicide. The plan calls for a coordinating committee, made up of members of relevant agencies in the community, which designates a host agency to take the lead role. Of key importance, institution of the plan should not be delayed until it is needed. It must be immediately available when a suicide cluster is occurring or seems about to occur, or when one or more deaths from trauma occur in the community, particularly among adolescents, which may influence others to attempt suicide (CDC 1988). Other elements of the plan include responding to the suicides in a manner that avoids glorification of the suicide victims and minimizes sensationalism; identifying other persons who may be at high risk of suicide, conducting at least one screening interview, and making referrals to counseling or other services as necessary; establishing agency spokespersons and providing a timely flow of accurate, appropriate information to the media; identifying and changing aspects of the environment that might increase the likelihood of further suicides or attempts; and addressing long-term issues suggested by the nature of the suicide cluster.

Even without a formal suicide-prevention committee, state and local agencies can work together to prevent suicide. Toll-free hot lines and walk-in counseling centers may help prevent some suicides and provide an entry point into the mental health system, but their effect on reducing the suicide rate appears to be small (National Committee for Injury Prevention and Control 1989). Working with hospitals and emergency medical services, local schools and universities, churches, parent groups, police, and the media, agencies can educate the public to recognize the warning signs of suicide and to know what to do when faced with a suicidal person or suicidal feelings. The state of California has developed an intensive program to train and license people to present a two-day suicide-intervention program to adolescents. Agency personnel are an obvious choice to participate in such a program or to develop and implement a similar program. Programs for survivors—those who have lost a close friend or relative to suicide—are considered important aspects of suicide prevention (those who survive suicide are three times more likely to complete suicide compared with the normal population [Dunne-Maxim 1986]). Agencies can be instrumental in starting survivor groups or offering other counseling to survivors.

Alcohol abuse, both acute and chronic, has been found to play a role in youth suicide (Brent et al. 1987). Measures to help young people combat alcohol abuse might also help prevent youth suicide. Agency personnel should be aware of the relationship between suicide and alcohol abuse, which may influence preventive measures for either or both conditions (e.g., alcohol abuse may cause depression, which is a risk factor for suicide [Brent et al. 1987]). Protective-service personnel must also be trained to recognize the signs and symptoms of suicide (see section 14.A) and must be alert to the fact that youth suicide may be a consequence of an abusive family.

Agencies can implement or advocate measures to reduce the availability of some common methods of committing suicide—for example, firearms (CDC 1988). Aspects of the environment that permit or encourage suicide should be modified, and sites where suicides have taken place should be immediately changed if possible to remove the hazard. For example, barriers should be erected to prevent suicides from cliffs, bridges, buildings, or railroad tracks. Garages or other buildings where suicides were attempted or completed should be made inaccessible to the public or closely monitored or both (CDC 1988). Building codes that prevent falls may also prevent suicide by jumping (Baker and Dietz 1979) (see chapter 10).

14.C.4 Legislators and Regulators

Statutes making suicide a criminal act are no longer common in the United States. Such statutes, which existed until recently, were not effective in preventing suicide but only served to add to the stigma surrounding suicide and hamper treatment efforts. Several other means of reducing youth suicide are available to federal, state, and local legislatures. Many states have passed legislation pertaining to youth suicide. For example, in 1983, the California legislature mandated a three-year youth suicide-prevention school program, which, at the end of two years, had resulted in significant gains in the understanding of prevention techniques among those high school students who completed a four-hour training course (Nelson 1987).

Regulating the sale of firearms, particularly handguns, (one study found that almost 70% of the firearms used in suicides were handguns [Wintemute et al. 1988]) should help limit access to guns and therefore reduce the incidence of suicide (Rivara 1983–1985) (see section 12.C.4). Alcohol has been found to play an important role in some suicides, especially suicides committed with firearms (Brent et al. 1987). Regulations that restrict minors' access to alcohol may help to prevent some suicides.

14.C.5 Law Enforcement Professionals

Law enforcement officers, like other professionals who interact with children and adolescents, need to be sensitive to the warning signs for suicide (see section 14.A). Youths in custody who exhibit suicidal behavior should be referred immediately for counseling. Belts and other objects that could be used for suicide by hanging should be removed, medications controlled, and the youths should be supervised closely (CDC 1988). If a suicidal child is at home, the family can be advised to limit access to weapons.

Enforcement officers are an integral part of a community suicide-prevention plan. Police might help locate desperate persons calling a suicide hot line, for instance (CDC 1988). Departmental policy can be developed such that, in the event of a suicide or suicide attempt, department spokespersons provide timely and accurate reports to the media, without embellishments. For example, they may say that an individual committed suicide by carbon monoxide poisoning, but not say the individual hooked up a garden hose to the exhaust of a car (CDC 1988). Providing operational details may make imitative suicide easier and therefore more likely.

Police efforts to alter or monitor environments where a suicide or suicide attempt occurred can help prevent future attempts. Strict enforcement of regulations restricting firearms and alcohol may help prevent some suicides.

The perpetrator may attempt to disguise a homicide by fabricating a history and arranging a scene to suggest suicide. Therefore, any apparent suicide should be investigated initially as a homicide. Presently, police departments are training personnel to recognize the signs of satanic worship and other cult behavior that may lead to human injury as part of ritual and may attract even early adolescents.

14.C.6 Voluntary Organizations

Children kill themselves after becoming hopeless. For any of a number of reasons or a combination of reasons, their family and community have failed to provide them with adequate emotional and social support to feel loved and connected. They have turned their aggression inward. Organized activities that aid families and prevent social isolation should be of general assistance. Support groups which help parents understand the emotional needs of children, which increase parenting skills and child-parent communication, and which assist families in dealing with grief should be of help. Adults who interact with children must take talk of suicide and suicidal behavior seriously and intervene to assure timely assessment by a mental health professional.

It is clear that young people who are suicidal are more likely to die if they have access to a gun (Brent et al. 1988). Community initiatives which decrease access to guns will decrease the number of suicides.

Copycat suicides within a community may sometimes be eliminated by modifying or eliminating the site of the first suicide.

14.C.7 Designers, Architects, Builders, and Engineers

Environmental changes can decrease intentional injury. When coal gas was eliminated as a fuel source in homes in Great Britain, the overall suicide rate decreased, as a result of a large decline in suicide by domestic gas (Kreitman 1976). Suicide patterns can be monitored for potential design changes which make lethal injury more difficult. Blister (individual-dose) packaging for medications and containers which hold a small total dose of drug are one such possibility; firearm design changes are another (see section 12.C.7).

14.C.8 Business and Industry

Over-the-counter drugs are often used in suicide gestures and suicides. Decreasing the total dose available to children or young adolescents whose suicidal acts often are impulsive, would be expected to decrease deaths. This can be accomplished by blister packaging which makes unwrapping a large number of pills or capsules extremely tedious or by packaging such preparations in containers which hold less than a lethal dose.

Purchasers of weapons can be encouraged to make them inaccessible to children and adolescents by either locking mechanisms or storage procedures.

Employee assistance programs may help prevent suicide by providing counseling services to employees or their family members who are at high risk.

14.C.9 Mass Media

People who attempt to influence others by making a suicide gesture may actually kill themselves if they are mistaken in their judgment of their weapon. A particularly clear example is that of deaths resulting from liver toxicity among those who initially recover from taking large amounts of acetaminophen, thinking it relatively benign (compared with aspirin, for instance) (Gazzard et al. 1976). Media warnings about drug side effects can influence doctors and parents, as exemplified by the rapid dissemination of information about the reputed association between aspirin and Reye Syndrome and the subsequent adoption of acetaminophen as the treatment of choice for fever or pain in children. More media attention to the liver toxicity from acetaminophen might prevent some suicide gestures from becoming suicides.

Whether publicity following a suicide, especially suicide by a person who has been admired or can be romanticized, precipitates imitative suicides is still being debated (Holinger 1990). An epidemic of suicides appeared to follow Goethe's publication of *The Sorrows of Young Werther*, so this is often called the "Werther effect." Studies of child suicide, a relatively rare occurrence, do not yet address this issue, but one might expect young adolescents to be as susceptible to imitative suicide as their older counterparts (Gould and Shaffer 1986; Phillips and Carstensen 1986). These imitative suicides may not be committed by people who would eventually kill themselves anyway and merely do so at an earlier time because of the publicized suicide; in other words, they may be additional and unnecessary deaths.

Although suicide is newsworthy, there are options as to how intensively and with what detail suicides are publicized. Certainly, curtailing the reporting of adolescent suicides and suicide attempts or avoiding the subject in fiction might be criticized as limiting the important right of free speech. On the other hand, discouraging gratuitous attention to adolescent suicide and the portrayal of suicide in general is worth discussing, as are the role and responsibility of the purveyor in developing and evaluating approaches to anticipating and preventing unfortunate consequences. The communications industry might develop a consensus code of ethics around this issue.

Televised programs about teen suicide sometimes are followed immediately by announcements about resources for help for those who are contemplating suicide. Whether or not such strategies are effective awaits evaluation, as does the contribution the media might make in advising the public about mental health and mental health services in general.

References

Baker, SP, and Dietz, PE. 1979. Injury Prevention. From *Healthy People, The Surgeon General's Report on Health Promotion and Disease Prevention*, Background Papers. Washington, D.C.: U.S. Dept. of Health, Education, and Welfare.

Beck, AT, et al. 1974. Development of suicidal intent scales, in Beck, AT, et al. (eds.): *The Prediction of Suicide*. Bowie, Md.: Charles Press Publishers, pp. 45-56.

Brent, DA. 1989. Suicide and suicidal behavior in children and adolescents. *Pediatr Rev* 10(9):269.

Brent, DA, et al. 1988. Risk factors for adolescent suicide: A comparison of adolescent suicide victims with suicidal inpatients. *Arch Gen Psychiatry* 45:581-588.

Brent, DA, et al. 1987. Alcohol, firearms, and suicide among youth: Temporal trends in Allegheny County, Pennsylvania, 1960 to 1983. *JAMA* 257(24): 3369-3372.

Centers for Disease Control. 1988. CDC recommendations for a community plan

for the prevention and containment of suicide clusters. *MMWR* 37(S-6):1-12.
Dunne-Maxim, K. 1986. Survivors of suicide. *J Psychosoc Nurs Ment Health Serv* 24(12):31-35.
Gazzard, BG, et al. 1976. Why do people use paracetamol for suicide? *Br Med J* 1:212-213.
Gould, MS, and Shaffer, D. 1986. The impact of suicide in television movies: Evidence of imitation. *N Engl J Med* 315(11):690-694.
Harkavy Friedman, JM, et al. 1987. Prevalence of specific suicidal behaviors in a high school sample. *Am J Psychiatry* 144:1203-1206.
Hawton, K. 1982. Attempted suicide in children and adolescents. *J Child Psychol Psychiatry* 23(4):497-503.
Hibbard, RA, et al. 1988. Abuse, feelings, and health behaviors in a student population. *Am J Dis Child* 142:326-330.
Holinger, PC. 1990. The causes, impact, and preventability of childhood injuries in the United States: Childhood suicide in the United States. *Am J Dis Child* 144:670-676.
Kreitman, N. 1976. The coal gas story: United Kingdom suicide rates, 1960-71. *Brit J Prev Soc Med* 30:86-93.
Lourie, RS. 1967. Suicide and attempted suicide in children and adolescents. *Texas Med* 63:58-63.
National Committee for Injury Prevention and Control. 1989. *Injury Prevention: Meeting the Challenge*. New York: Oxford University Press.
Nelson, FL. 1987. Evaluation of a youth suicide prevention school program. *Adolescence* 22(88):813-825.
Orbach, I. 1986. The "insolvable problem" as a determinant in the dynamics of suicidal behavior in children. *Am J Psychother* 40(4):511-520.
Orbach, I. 1988. *Children Who Don't Want to Live*. San Francisco: Jossey-Bass.
Otto, U. 1972. Suicidal acts by children and adolescents: A follow-up study. *Acta Psychiatr Scand Suppl* 233:7-123.
Phillips, DP, and Carstensen, LL. 1986. Clustering of teenage suicides after television news stories about suicide. *N Engl J Med* 315(11):685.
Rivara, FP. 1983-1985. Epidemiology of violent deaths in children and adolescents in the United States. *Pediatrician* 12(1):3-10.
Rosenthal, P, and Rosenthal, S. 1984. Suicidal behaviors by preschool children. *Am J Psychiatry* 141(4):520-525.
Ross, CP, and Lee, AR. N.d. *Suicide in Youth and What You Can Do about It: A Guide for School Personnel*. Burlingame, Calif.: Suicide Prevention and Crisis Center of San Mateo County.
Shaw, KR, et al. 1987. Suicide in children and adolescents. *Adv Pediatr* 34:313-334.
Smith, K, and Crawford, S. 1986. Suicidal behavior among "normal" high school students. *Suicide Life Threat Behav* 16(3):313-325.
Trinkoff, AM, and Baker, SP. 1986. Poisoning hospitalizations and deaths from solids and liquids among children and teenagers. *Am J Pubic Health* 76(6):657-660.
Weisman, AD, and Worden, JW. 1972. Risk-rescue rating in suicide assessment. *Arch Gen Psychiat* 26:553-560.
Wintemute, GJ, et al. 1988. The choice of weapons in firearm suicides. *Am J Public Health* 78(7):824-826.

Additional Sources of Information

American Academy of Child and Adolescent Psychiatry
3615 Wisconsin Avenue, NW
Washington, DC 20016
202-966-7300
   Information on youth suicide.

American Association of Suicidology (AAS)
2459 South Ash
Denver, CO, 80222
303-692-0985
   Information and resources on youth suicide.

American Psychological Association (APA)
1200 Seventeenth Street, NW
Washington, DC 20036
202-955-7673
   Information on youth suicide.

Youth Suicide National Center
1825 Eye Street, NW
Suite 400
Washington, DC 20006
   Materials for teachers and for students; technical assistance and training available for schools and agencies establishing programs.

IV

THE SCHOOL AND RECREATION ENVIRONMENT

15

Playground Injuries

15.A Facts

Traditional playgrounds, with their predictable pieces of equipment (swings, slides, climbers, seesaws, merry-go-rounds), have a small and somewhat age-limited role in children's play. On the other hand, an estimated 170,000 injuries associated with playground equipment prompt emergency room treatment each year (CPSC 1989). Rates for males and females are similar. Almost all the injured are children younger than 12, and more than 3,600 are hospitalized. Deaths do occur, often from head injury resulting from falls from swings, slides, and climbers. The most severe injuries usually involve falls from high equipment, strangulation, or entrapment of part of the body.

More than half the injuries, including about 90% of serious injuries, occur when a child falls or jumps from equipment to the surface below it. The most common serious injury is fracture of the forearm. Injuries of the head and face are also common. There are modest differences among the injury patterns for public playground equipment, home playground equipment (mostly "swing sets"), and homemade equipment (mostly tree swings). The majority of the reported injuries are incurred on public playground equipment (70%), often in school yards and public parks. There, not surprisingly, the average age of children injured is somewhat older than those injured at home, and the injuries are most likely to involve climbing equipment, followed by slides and swings, whereas falls from swings make up the largest group of injuries involving home and homemade equipment. Falls from public playground equipment that result in injury tend to be from a greater height than those from home equipment, though in both locations most falls are from heights under 8 feet. Slides are associated with falls of greater heights than other equipment (CPSC 1978).

The type of surface a child falls on, particularly its ability to absorb energy (impact attenuation), affects the likelihood of injury. Specially designed or prepared protective surfaces are superior to natural surfaces like dirt and grass, and natural surfaces, in turn, are superior to pavement (see section 15.C.7). Choosing and maintaining surfacing to diminish the likelihood of injury—especially head injury—is of prime importance to playground safety. Barriers and other design features which preclude falls from heights are a second obvious solution.

Some severe injuries and deaths involve strangulation by hanging in ropes or chains or when clothing becomes caught on a protrusion, entrapment of a finger or the head in a small space or angle, or impact with moving equipment or from collapsing equipment.

The siting of equipment in relation to likely activity paths is important so that children do not collide and are not tempted to run behind swings, in front of sliding boards, or into the path of bicyclists or motorists. Moving equipment that can strike children, such as swing seats, should be of designs and materials that will inflict as little damage as possible. Children on the playground and traveling to and from the playground should be protected from vehicular traffic.

Further details are provided in section 15.C.7. General guidelines for new and existing playgrounds are presented in Volume 1 of the Consumer Product Safety Commission's *Handbook for Public Playground Safety* (CPSC 1981a). Technical guidelines are detailed in Volume 2 (CPSC 1981b).

15.B Developmental Considerations

Play, though difficult to define precisely, appears to be crucial to normal childhood development. Among characteristics generally ascribed to play are activity, spontaneity, fun, purposelessness, and self-initiation (Frost and Klein 1983). Play is closely linked to exploratory behaviors and learning and may be a necessary part of socialization. As children develop, they acquire increasingly sophisticated and social forms of play, although they do not completely abandon earlier forms.

Perfectly normal play may pose a risk of injury, as many of the chapters in this book describe. Children play with all interesting and useful objects, not confining themselves to adult-defined "toys." Likewise, they explore and play in diverse environments, many of which are dangerous. Relatively little of a child's total play experience takes place on a "playground." In fact, formal playgrounds are a postindustrialization phenomenon, and the typical U.S. school playground — with swings, slide, climber, seesaws, and merry-go-round, set over asphalt — is a post–World War II development (Frost and Klein 1983). Such playgrounds foster only a limited range of play, as the following age-related descriptions suggest. It is particularly difficult to meet the needs of children of different ages with such a playground, and when the playground is shared by children of different ages, its dangers are probably increased.

An additional important developmental consideration in the design of playground equipment is the size of children of the age for which the equipment is intended. A compendium of average measurements for body parts of children of both sexes is available (Snyder et al. 1979).

15.B.1 Infants

Play begins in infancy with simple actions which are repeated apparently first for mastery and then for pleasure. This earliest form of play to appear is called *functional play*. It reappears often throughout childhood when a new skill is practiced. A 5-month-old infant who is mouthing and shaking a rattle over and over again is engaging in functional play, as is a 6-year-old who attempts to walk the length of a curb without falling.

Because infants are not yet independently mobile and playgrounds emphasize large-muscle skills, infants are passive participants on playgrounds. They love the rhythmic motion of the swing, for instance, but their safety will depend on the quality of the equipment and surfacing as well as the wisdom and presence of their parent or caregiver. For example, infant swings must not allow the child to fall out. The swing should be close to the ground. The surface below should be forgiving. Areas for infant play should be widely separated from the play of older children and from flying and moving equipment.

15.B.2 Toddlers

Toward the end of the second year, children put together play materials to create something new — a block building, a painting, a clay cookie — in what is called *construction play*. Like functional play, most children continue to engage in construction play.

Throughout infancy and toddlerhood, play is often "solitary," that is, the child's play is not interactive. It does not involve other children. Even when the child begins to play "with" another child by the age of $2\frac{1}{2}$ or 3, the play may be "parallel" rather than interactive; the children play alongside one another without significant interaction.

Because of their enchantment with learning to walk, run, and climb, most toddlers are delighted by the playground. On the other hand, it holds almost endless injury possibilities for the short, slow, unsteady toddler who has no judgment and is mixing with and mimicking older children. Where heights and moving equipment cannot be avoided, an adult must be at the toddler's side and a soft surface below.

15.B.3 Preschoolers

Three-, four-, and five-year-olds exhibit increasingly sophisticated forms of *symbolic play*, of which make-believe is the defining characteristic. Objects, places, and situations are imagined. In its most advanced form, symbolic play is *sociodramatic*, with children taking different roles by agreement. Playing "house" and "cops and robbers" are two examples.

Likewise, the preschooler moves from the parallel play of toddlerhood through "associative" play (from about ages $3\frac{1}{2}$ to $4\frac{1}{2}$), sharing materials and activities with other children, into truly "cooperative" play which requires group organization. Preschoolers do not cooperate consistently, however, in ways that would protect them from injury on the playground. They cannot be depended upon to take turns, to stay out of the way, or to anticipate injury risks to themselves or their playmates. Quite the opposite is true. Their developmental drive to try new roles, behaviors, and skills can be counted on to put them at risk. They will push and shove, climb and fall. Physics is completely beyond them. They do not make time and space calculations before they run behind the swing or think about velocity when they get off a moving merry-go-round. They dismount from the seesaw without notice and let their companion fall. No amount of lecturing will produce safe playground behavior.

15.B.4 Elementary School Ages

Only at about age 6 does a child begin to play *games with rules*, also a form of cooperative play. Most sports fall under this play rubric. Games with rules differ from sociodramatic play not only by having rules, but also by their emphasis on skills and competition (Frost and Klein 1983). The school-age child continues, of course, to engage in the prior forms of play, and to look for new challenges. Children's increasing abilities, their drive to be "first" and "best," and their desire for peer approval lead them to be daring on the playground—to see who can jump farthest from the swing, who can climb the highest, who can come down the slide fastest and in the most unusual position. Thrills are the name of the game, and injuries are inevitable if protection is not built in.

15.B.5 Young Adolescents

While the "play" of the young adolescent falls into the categories outlined, several aspects deserve special comment. Many young adolescents spend time practicing for and competing in games which emphasize skills (e.g., sports, which are covered in chapter 16). They mimic the games of adults and produce predictable patterns of injury. Young adolescents assume increasingly adultlike recreational roles and attempt adult skills which they have not mastered. Peer pressure is strong. For some, play includes the deliberate taking of risk, particularly to impress their friends.

15.C Opportunities for Protection

STRATEGIES FOR PREVENTING PLAYGROUND INJURIES
(High-priority strategies are indicated by a △).

Preventing Falls
  Provide handrails or guardrails for steps and platforms.
  Ensure that surfaces are slip-resistant under wet and dry conditions.

Reducing the Force of a Fall

△ Replace concrete and asphalt under play equipment with energy-absorbing materials.

Limit the height of playground equipment or the potential fall distance.

Eliminating or Reducing Other Hazards

△ Remove protrusions that could injure a falling child or snag clothing and lead to strangulation.

△ Design equipment with spaces and angles that preclude entrapment.

△ Avoid use of trampolines, gliders, and merry-go-rounds.

Arrange moving equipment such as swings so that children on foot are unlikely to be struck.

Replace metal or wooden swing seats with energy-absorbing materials.

Remove particularly dangerous equipment from playgrounds.

Ensure frequent maintenance of equipment and surfaces.

Separate playgrounds from motor vehicle and bicycle traffic.

Provide safe pedestrian and bicycle routes to public playgrounds.

15.C.1 Schools and Child Care Centers

Playground injuries are the leading school injury category for elementary school students (Sheps and Evans 1987) and are also experienced by children at day care centers. The greatest opportunity for schools and child care centers to reduce the number and severity of playground injuries is in modifying the design of the playground itself rather than in modifying the behavior of children. Many playgrounds present obvious hazards. The playground should be thought of as the workplace of children, and efforts should be made to provide as safe a workplace as possible. Materials are available to educate teachers and day care personnel in playground safety (see additional sources of information).

It is wholly foreseeable that children on playground equipment will slip, fall, push each other, and otherwise act with little regard for safety. The punishment for acting as children should not be serious injury. The playground equipment, layout, and surfaces should be chosen so that forces in anticipated falls, collisions, etc., are distributed over the body in a forgiving and noninjurious manner. This can be achieved with rounded edges and smooth, yielding surfaces.

Schools and child care centers should provide play areas geared to the developmental stages of the children they serve. Play areas for young children should be separated from those for older children. Playgrounds should be designed to provide at least the protections accorded by CPSC guidelines and the recommendations discussed in section 15.C.7. Existing playgrounds should be reviewed for safety conditions. Equipment deemed hazardous due to design or layout should be removed. Hard surfacing under equipment should be removed and replaced with safer surfacing.

Playgrounds for preschoolers should be protected by fencing at least 4 feet high; if the playground is on a roof, the fence should be 7 feet high (CWLA 1984). Comfortable seating near popular equipment or play areas encourages close adult supervision (AAP 1987).

Day care and school systems should have written policies detailing playground layout and design, supervisory duties, playground rules, emergency procedures, injury-reporting procedures, and routine playground maintenance. A playground safety checklist should be adapted for each particular playground and checked as part of routine maintenance. Records of injuries occurring on playgrounds should be routinely collected and maintained. Review and analysis of these records should be made by trained persons to determine high-risk equipment and activities. Modifications of equipment and activities should be made on the basis of these findings. Schools serving handicapped children should modify the existing playground or develop new play areas accessible to all. Playground rules and procedures should be taught to students in the beginning of the school year and reinforced as necessary.

15.C.2 Health Care Providers

Child care facilities and schools often have health care providers as advisors on child health matters. Since most will have or plan some kind of a playground, professionals serving in this capacity should make playground safety a high priority. Particularly important is the opportunity to assure that the structures and surfaces are chosen with safety in mind.

For preschoolers, playground injuries occur most frequently on home equipment (CDC 1988). The health care provider may be the only informed professional who has access to the parents to advise them during the stage of the child's development when they are considering playground equipment for home use. Counseling points might well include installation over energy-absorbing surfaces, locating equipment away from other objects, adequate anchoring, and the immediate repair or removal of broken equipment (CDC 1988). Trampolines should be discouraged for home playgrounds for children of all ages.

15.C.3 Public Agencies

Community and urban planners need to provide play areas for children. In public housing, for instance, studies have shown that the suitability of the environment for children and children's play strongly influences residents' satisfaction with the housing (Coyle 1980). Play areas should be accessible to children with handicaps.

Agencies should establish criteria for the design of safe playgrounds and the selection of safe playground equipment; procedures for routine inspection and maintenance of children's play areas at public housing sites, parks, and schools; and procedures for inspection and enforcement at private schools, child care centers, and day care homes. Some design recommendations are presented in section 15.C.7. Playgrounds should conform at least to the CPSC guidelines discussed there. Checklists, handbooks, and videotapes are available, and playground inspection services are available if manpower or expertise is lacking (see additional sources of information). Risk-management systems ensure that the challenges necessarily provided by playgrounds do not result in injury and minimize the exposure to liability (Bruya and Beckwith 1985-1986; Moore et al. 1987). Telephones should be available near playgrounds to call for help when an injury has occurred. Ponds and other bodies of water should be inaccessible to unsupervised children.

It is possible to design safe play areas that are as much fun as risky ones. Resources are available to help agencies work with communities to rehabilitate existing playgrounds (Regenbogen 1981); to build new playgrounds from scrap and donated materials (Frost and Klein 1983); to identify underutilized spaces and develop them as play areas (Klein and Sears 1980); and to enlist parents to serve as supervisors at children's play areas (Gustafsson et al. 1979).

Playgrounds should be safely accessible to children, separated from motor vehicle traffic. Attractive bicycle-riding paths should be provided so bicyclists do not ride in the play area. Traffic and warning signs that children can understand should be posted. Children are unlikely to use play areas that are distant from their daily lives; the street and sidewalk in front of their homes are popular alternatives for many. The impact on injury of designated "people streets"—streets intended for use by people, not vehicles—has not been established. Interested agencies could explore this alternative—identifying qualifying streets, encouraging residents to apply for the designation, restricting all or some motor vehicle traffic, making designated streets more suitable for recreation, and evaluating the results (Baltimore Department of Planning 1977).

Vandalism and litter can be ongoing problems that make playgrounds not only unattractive but also unsafe. Countermeasures include making the playground more visible from the street to allow for surveillance; providing security lighting to all areas of the facility; and working with neighborhood groups to encourage maintenance. "Bottle bills," which promote return of glass containers, have been effective in reducing glass-related lacerations in children (Baker et al. 1986) and may reduce the amount of broken glass on playground surfaces, making the least-expensive energy-absorbing materials, such as sand or wood chips, which might hide pieces of glass, a more viable alternative.

15.C.4 Legislators and Regulators

Guidelines for playground safety, exemplified by the Consumer Product Safety Commission's *Handbook for Public Playground Safety* (CPSC 1981a, 1981b), are helpful but have been criticized on a number of points, including being limited to conventional public playground equipment (Frost 1985-1986) and a lack of attention to surfacing needs. They are, for the most part, suggested design standards, and they have no force of law. Development of detailed performance standards which focus on hazards rather than specific pieces of equipment and are aimed at both normal use patterns and foreseeable misuse has been suggested as a progressive direction (Wilkinson 1985-1986) and is more consonant with the accepted regulatory approach.

"Bottle bills" requiring deposit and return of glass and plastic containers might help reduce broken glass and litter at playgrounds (Baker et al. 1986). Zoning regulations of municipalities can require that new residential developments provide play areas that are removed from traffic and that are easily and safely accessible to children.

15.C.5 Law Enforcement Professionals

The presence of law enforcement personnel patrolling parks and playgrounds discourages criminal acts which may lead to injury (such as littering and violence) and increases enforcement of state and local ordinances. Curfew laws exist in some communities; they work best when strictly enforced.

15.C.6 Voluntary Organizations

Organizations that use or provide playground and playing facilities for recreational programs should make provisions to assure that the equipment and surfaces are in good repair. Regular, structured inspections should be carried out in order to avoid not only injuries but also liability. Persons responsible for playgrounds have been found negligent for not providing an energy-absorbing surface when children have been injured in falls (Sweeney 1987).

15.C.7 Designers, Architects, Builders, and Engineers

Traditional American public playgrounds do not promote a full range of play (see section 15.B), appear to be underutilized, are often installed and then poorly maintained, and may be unsafe not only because the equipment or surface is hazardous but also because they can become the site of child misuse or drug dealing. Playground designs should attract children of an appropriate age. They should promote safe, interesting, and creative play on equipment that is easy to maintain, resists destruction with use, lasts well, and is installed over a surface which minimizes injury if a child falls. Playgrounds should be accessible to children with handicaps, such as those in wheelchairs or visually impaired. Attention should be given not only to design within the playground but also to location. Locations near homes

Table 15-1. G-Forces Recorded for Test Object Dropped from Various Heights onto Different Playground Surfacing Materials

Surface Material in Inches	Drop Height in Feet				
	$\frac{1}{2}$	1	2	4	8
Wet packed sand, 10	–	–	–	–	10–13
Wood chips, 12	–	–	–	–	30–35
Pea gravel, 8	–	–	10–15	–	15–40
Rubber mat, $1\frac{1}{8}$	–	3–5	6–15	40–55	–
Packed earth	–	–	–	175–225	–
Asphalt	60–65	140–160	–	–	–
Concrete	250–300	475–525	–	–	–

Adapted from CPSC 1976.

Note: The threshold for serious head injury is thought to be about 50 Gs and for fatalities about 160 Gs.

and streets appear to be the most utilized, but barriers between the play area and traffic must be assured. Traffic encounters on the way to and from the playground should also be considered (RoSPA 1987). Comfortable seating for adults should be provided near popular equipment or play areas. Lighting should ensure visibility from the street and in all parts of the park, for security.

Public and home playground designs should take into account the safety of individual pieces of equipment during use and foreseeable misuse (see CPSC 1981a and 1981b for design guidelines), prevention of falls from heights, the energy-absorbing characteristics of the surface under and around the equipment (see table 15-1), spacing of the equipment, and adequate separation of play areas intended for different purposes (Goldberger 1987). Prevention of hanging from entrapment of the head or clothing and the ease of installation and maintenance must also be considered. Designs for playground equipment for home use should be approached with the same care as for public playgrounds. Specifics include the following (Wilkinson 1985–1986):

- Materials and surface finishes should be selected for their durability and resistance to deterioration; finishes should be nontoxic.
- Equipment should be constructed to withstand static- or dynamic-load testing and to withstand maximum anticipated forces tending to tip the equipment when properly installed.
- Hardware should be strong.
- Sharp edges or surfaces, pinch and crush points, and protrusions should be avoided.
- Suspended elements (e.g., swing seats) should be made of materials that minimize force, such as canvas.
- The velocity of rotating equipment should be controlled by design, and safe exit assured.

- Slide inclines and exits should minimize exit velocity.
- There should be no openings that can trap a child's head.
- High equipment (more than 2.5 m) should have enclosed top portions. Equipment of intermediate height should have effective guardrails.
- Ladders and railings should provide good gripping surfaces, and inclines and steps should be suitable for the intended users.
- Hard surfaces should be avoided under the equipment.

Handrails should be graspable and placed at the correct height for children. Guardrails for platforms and equipment should be spaced to prevent children from falling through, to prevent head entrapment and to discourage climbing. Angles less than 55 degrees should be avoided to prevent head or extremity entrapment. Surfaces should be slip-resistant under wet and dry conditions. The height that a child falls from a sliding board can be reduced by building the slide into a hill or onto a pyramidal structure (see figure 15-1). A child's speed on a sliding board is determined by the height, surface, friction, and slope; an average slope of no more than 30 degrees is recommended.

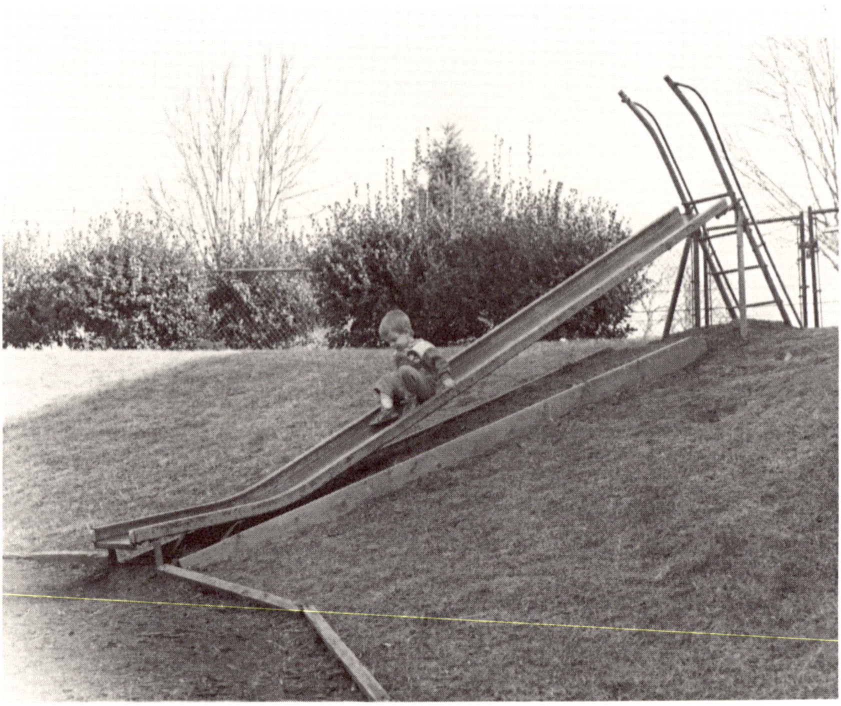

FIGURE 15-1. *Slide built over a hill minimizes the height of a fall. The railing shown under this slide may cause injury in a fall and should be removed.*

Because impact with gliders causes many injuries (CPSC 1979), gliders might be omitted from swing sets. Trampolines have been associated with very disabling injuries and should not be provided on public or private playgrounds.

Labeling should warn the purchaser of the dangers of installing playground equipment over hard surfacing (Sweeney 1979). Concrete and asphalt paving should not be used, and dirt often becomes packed so hard that it does not absorb the energy of a fall. Loose materials such as sand, wood chips, and shredded tires help to cushion a fall if they are deep enough but may lose some of their resilience when wet and require regular maintenance in order to remain effective as cushioning materials. Some resilient mats provide excellent energy attenuation when installed on level, uniform surfaces. The "forgiving" surface must extend beyond the equipment on all sides to the maximum distance a child might be thrown in a fall, a distance which varies by equipment type (Burke 1987).

15.C.8 Business and Industry

Manufacturers of playground equipment for public or home use should provide adequate instructions for installation, including surfacing of the site and spacing of equipment (Burke 1987), and for maintenance. Permanent labels should be affixed identifying the manufacturer and the age-group for which the equipment is designed (Wilkinson 1985–1986).

Premarket testing of new designs may help to avoid some injuries. Equipment associated with especially severe injuries should be voluntarily withdrawn. Certain pieces, trampolines might be one example, should not be marketed for general use.

15.C.9 Mass Media

Of all playground modifications to reduce injury, provision of a compressible surface under equipment is likely to have the most far-reaching beneficial effect. The media can popularize the concept of "forgiving" surfaces. Since many playground injuries occur at home, public awareness of the need for sturdy equipment which is properly installed and maintained is also crucial. The height of equipment should be emphasized, and innovative solutions can be shown, such as building slides into hill sides (see figure 15-1).

Investigative journalists might find the topic of playgrounds particularly fertile. Comparing local conditions to recommendations from the CPSC or other standards might lead to beneficial attention and change. Safer equipment and designs might also be brought to public attention this way. The opportunity for effective visuals is great.

Reduction in lacerations to children (Baker et al. 1986) and an increase in safety of playgrounds is a little-mentioned beneficial side effect of "bottle bills" which require deposits on glass containers. This aspect of the laws can be included in reporting on such legislative initiatives.

References

American Academy of Pediatrics. 1987. *Health in Day Care: A Manual for Health Professionals.* Elk Grove Village, Ill.: American Academy of Pediatrics.

Baker, MD, et al. 1986. The impact of "bottle bill" legislation on the incidence of lacerations in childhood. *Am J Public Health* 76(10):1243-1244.

Baltimore Department of Housing and Community Development. 1975. *Twelve Parks in Retrospect.* Baltimore: Dept. of Housing and Community Development.

Baltimore Department of Planning, Baltimore City Planning Commission. 1977. *The Design of Neighborhood Parks.* Baltimore: Dept. of Planning.

Bruya, LD, and Beckwith, J. 1985-1986. Due process: Reducing exposure to liability suits and the management risks associated with children's play areas. *Children's Environments Quarterly* 2(4):29.

Burke, W. 1987. Preventing playground injuries. *Park/Grounds Management* June: 6-7.

Centers for Disease Control. 1988. Playground-related injuries in preschool-aged children — United States, 1983-1987. *MMWR* 37(41):629-632.

Child Welfare League of America. 1984. *Standards for Day Care Service*, revised edition. New York: Child Welfare League of America.

Consumer Product Safety Commission. 1976. *Prepared Standard for Public Playground Equipment.* Washington, D.C.: Consumer Product Safety Commission.

Consumer Product Safety Commission. 1978. *Hazard Analysis: Injuries Associated with Public Playground Equipment.* Report prepared by G. Rutherford. Washington, D.C.: Consumer Product Safety Commission.

Consumer Product Safety Commission. 1979. *Home Playground Equipment Injuries Treated in Hospital Emergency Rooms—1978.* Report prepared by G. Rutherford. Washington, D.C.: Consumer Product Safety Commission.

Consumer Product Safety Commission. 1981a. *A Handbook for Public Playground Safety.* Vol. 1. *General Guidelines for New and Existing Playgrounds.* Washington, D.C.: Consumer Product Safety Commission.

Consumer Product Safety Commission. 1981b. *A Handbook for Public Playground Safety.* Vol. 2. *Technical Guidelines for Equipment and Surfacing.* Washington, D.C.: Consumer Product Safety Commission.

Consumer Product Safety Commission. 1987. *Preliminary NEISS Estimates of National Injuries.* Washington, D.C.: Consumer Product Safety Commission.

Consumer Product Safety Commission. 1989. *Playground Equipment-Related Injuries Involving Falls to the Surface.* Report prepared by DK Tinsworth and JT Kramer. Washington, D.C.: Consumer Product Safety Commission.

Coyle, T. 1980. *Incentives as an Aid for Improving the Quality of the Family Housing Environment: A Position Paper.* CEAS Research Project 20. Ottawa, Ontario: Canada Mortgage and Housing Corporation.

Frost, JL. 1985-1986. History of playground safety in America. *Children's Environments Quarterly* 2(4):13.

Frost, JL, and Klein, BL. 1983. *Children's Play and Playgrounds.* Austin, Tex.: Playgrounds International.

Goldberger, P. 1987. Great American playgrounds. *Child* 2(3):62.

Gustafsson, LH, et al. 1979. Child-environment supervisors: A new strategy for prevention of childhood accidents. *Acta Paediatr Scand* 275(suppl):102–107.

Klein and Sears Research, et al. 1980. *Lost and Found: Recycling Space for Children.* CEAS Research Project 8. Ottawa, Ontario: Canada Mortgage and Housing Corporation.

Larsson, NK. 1980. *The Nature of Child-Related Maintenance and Vandalism Problems in CMHC Family Housing Projects.* CEAS Research Project 3. Ottawa, Ontario: Canada Mortgage and Housing Corporation.

Moore, RC, et al. 1987. *Play for All Guidelines: Planning, Design and Management of Outdoor Play Settings for All Children.* Berkeley, Calif.: MIG Communications.

Regenbogen, T. 1981. *A Place to Share: How Your Neighbourhood May Help Itself, Its Children, Young People and Families.* CEAS Report. Ottawa, Ontario: Canada Mortgage and Housing Corporation.

Royal Society for the Prevention of Accidents. 1987. *Statement on Children's Play.* Birmingham, UK: Royal Society for the Prevention of Accidents.

Sheps, SB, and Evans, GD. 1987. Epidemiology of school injuries: A 2-year experience in a municipal health department. *Pediatrics* 79(1):69–75.

Snyder, RG, et al. 1979. *Anthropometry of Infants, Children, and Youths to Age 18 for Product Safety Design.* Warrendale, Pa.: Society of Automotive Engineers.

Sweeney, T. 1987. Playgrounds and head injuries: A problem for the school business manager. *School Business Affairs* 53(1):28–31.

Sweeney, T. 1979. Playground accidents: A new perspective. *Trial* 15(4):40–44.

Wilkinson, PF. 1985–1986. Safety in children's play environments. *Children's Environments Quarterly.* 2(4):9–12.

Additional Sources of Information

Association for Childhood Education International (ACEI)
11141 Georgia Avenue
Suite 200
Wheaton, MD 20902
800-423-3562
   Information for teachers on play, including a video on playground safety.

ASTM (formerly known as the American Society for Testing and Materials)
1916 Race Street
Philadelphia, PA 19103
215-299-5400
   Playground-surfacing standards.

Bergwall Productions
PO Box 238
Garden City, NY 11530
   Videos on playground safety for child care personnel.

Canada Mortgage and Housing Corporation (CMHC)
682 Montreal Road
Ottawa, Ontario K1A 0P7
Canada
613-748-2362
   Information on play spaces in the residential environment, including *An International Inventory and Comparative Study of Legislation and Guidelines for Children's Play Spaces in the Residential Environment.*

Canadian Institute of Child Health (CICH)
17 York Street
Suite 105
Ottawa, Ontario
Canada
613-238-8425
 Guidelines for playground safety (Canadian playground standards derived from these guidelines).

Consumer Product Safety Commission (CPSC)
5401 Westbard Avenue
Washington, DC 20207
800-638-CPSC or 301-492-6580
 Guidelines for playground safety.

Kompan Incorporated
80 King Spring Road
Windsor Locks, CT 06096
203-623-4139
 Information on playground equipment and various international standards, including *Comparison between Various Equipment Standards* (1984).

National Playing Fields Association (NPFA)
PO Box 55
Godmanchester, Huntington, Cambs. 188XF
UK
 Information on playground design and management; computerized bibliographic service.

PLAE, Inc. (Play and Learning in Adaptable Environments)
1824 A Fourth Street
Berkeley, CA 94710
415-845-7523
 Guidelines and other information on playground design incorporating injury prevention, risk management, and handicapped users; *Play for All News* newsletter.

Playground Clearinghouse
36 Sycamore Lane
Phoenixville, PA 19460
215-935-1549
 Information and consultation on playground safety, risk management, and inspections.

Recreation and Safety Institute (RSI)
PO Box 392
Ronkonkoma, NY 11779
516-563-4800
 Information on playground management, risk reduction, litigation and legislative trends; offers playground services and hazard identification video.

16

Sports Injuries

16.A Facts

This chapter addresses both organized sports such as school programs and informal sports such as skateboarding and backyard ball playing but excludes forms of recreation that are discussed in other chapters (see especially Playground Injuries, Drowning, Animals, Falls, Bicyclists, Users of Other Motor Vehicles).

Sports injuries are very common but have a low fatality rate. With the exception of the sports addressed in other chapters, sports-related fatalities are rare in the under-15 age-group. The CPSC identified an average of 12 deaths annually (CPSC 1981), with baseball causing the largest number and football the second largest. Given the low number of injuries associated with golf in general, the fact that it ranks third in number of deaths to 5- to 14-year-olds in organized sports is worthy of mention. Most deaths are due to blows to the head from a ball or club. Some victims are spectators. Trampolines have been associated with a number of deaths and permanent spinal cord injuries. On average, for each sports-related death there are about 50,000 injuries that require emergency room treatment.

The incidence of sports injuries is about twice as high for boys as for girls and increases with age; a sharp rise at about age 12 corresponds with the beginning of junior high school, when team sports become more prominent and competition sharpens. Team sports account for more than half of all sports injuries, with football, baseball, and basketball the leading causes (see table 16-1). The relative hazard of various sports is not clearly established, however, because of inadequate reporting of injury and lack of knowledge of the number of participants and the intensity of participation for many sports and forms of recreation (Kraus and Conroy 1984). Data are particularly poor for children. Estimates based on 1980 data put the number of medically treated injuries per thousand participants aged 5–14 for four team sports to be the following: football, 119; baseball, 75; basketball, 43; and ice hockey, 41 (CPSC 1981).

Although life-threatening injuries during sports and informal recreation usually result from excessive forces on the head, neck, or chest, many injuries are to the extremities. Unlike older adolescents and adults, for

Table 16-1. Estimated Number of Childhood Injuries Related to Selected Sports Treated in U.S. Emergency Rooms, Ages 0–14, 1987

Activity	Total Injuries	Activity	Total Injuries
Football	125,000	Track and field	9,800
Baseball	113,500	Scooters	9,000
Basketball	104,400	Skiing	8,700
Skateboarding	67,500	Weight lifting	8,500
Roller skating	44,200	Golf	7,700
Unspecified ball	42,000	Field hockey	6,700
Soccer	36,100	Ice skating	6,200
Gymnastics	22,600	Racketball/tennis	4,800
Fishing	22,200	Ice hockey	3,400
Sledding	21,600	Skating, unspecified	2,800
Volleyball	18,500	Bowling	2,600
Wrestling	12,600	Horseshoes	1,300
Trampoline	10,700		

Source: 1987 National Electronic Injury Surveillance System (NEISS) data from CPSC.

Note: Excludes injuries related to water sports, guns, bicycles, horseback riding, playground equipment, and motor vehicles, which are discussed in other chapters. Numbers rounded to nearest 100.

whom lower-extremity injuries make up the greatest proportion of injuries in team sports, child participants are more likely to injure their hand or arm, except in soccer, where ankle and knee injuries predominate (CPSC 1981). Little is known about the rate of long-term disability for either type of injury.

Deaths among young baseball players result from blows to the head by bats and baseballs or from blows to the chest, which can lead to cardiac arrest. Batting helmets and chest protection are therefore important protective measures. Dramatic reductions in injuries to the knee, ankle, etc., caused by sliding into fixed bases have resulted from the use of "breakaway" bases that yield on impact.

Football-related injuries to the head and neck are of special concern because of the potential for long-term consequences. Spearing and face tackling are no longer permitted in organized games because they use the head as a primary contact point. Concussions (brain injury from a blow to the head) represent about 3% of all football injuries (Listernick and Finison 1983); a player who is suspected to have received a concussion should not be returned to play in the same game (see section 16.C.2). Knee injuries, which are common and often lead to disability, can be reduced by preseason conditioning.

Face protection for ice hockey players, mouth guards for football players, and eye protection for children playing squash or other racquet sports have been shown to reduce many of the injuries that result when players are struck by balls, equipment, or other players. Well-designed protective helmets can absorb the energy of a blow to the head of horseback riders, whose most serious risk is of head injury (see chapter 12), and of participants in high-speed recreational activities such as skateboarding and ski racing.

Skateboarding and skiing also exemplify the importance of the environment. Surface irregularities play a major role in causing skateboarding and roller skating injuries. In the case of skiing, grooming ski slopes and removing or padding fixed obstacles has contributed to injury reduction. Similarly, protrusions from gymnasium walls should be removed, and the walls themselves padded in areas where athletes may run into them. In football and other field sports, a wide buffer zone should be established between the playing field and benches or other furniture that players could run into. These strategies illustrate general principles that can be applied to the prevention of injuries in virtually all sports.

In choosing among sports and in determining the degree to which children should be protected against injury, freedom from serious injury should be the objective. Minor cuts and superficial injury without lasting consequences are a small price to pay for the fun and learning associated with both formal and informal sports. Disabling injuries to the brain, spinal cord, internal organs, and joints, on the other hand, deserve attention and remedies wherever possible.

16.B Developmental Considerations

16.B.1 Infants

Babies do not, of course, participate in organized competitive sports. Though motor development is a major theme of infancy, its progression appears to be driven largely by the programmed development of the nervous and musculoskeletal systems. Infants need only be provided with attractive environments which stimulate their curiosity and provide safe arenas for their natural drive to independence and control. Though infant exercise programs are popular with some parents, there is no evidence that they contribute to the attainment of advanced or superior motor skills (AAP 1988a). The musculoskeletal system of the infant is probably particularly vulnerable to injury, and movement should not be forced. Infants and toddlers brought to view sporting events should be kept well away from the field of play so that they are not struck by equipment or players and should be protected from excessive sun exposure.

16.B.2 and 16.B.3 Toddlers and Preschoolers

Growing children explore not only their surroundings but also the roles they observe. When they see older children and adults they admire participating in sports, they may very well imitate their movements and expressions. They may enjoy trying to hit a big ball with a fat plastic bat or kicking a wobbling football along the ground. They do not yet possess the refined motor and judgment skills necessary to perform sporting activities at all well nor to protect themselves from injury. The period of time they are likely to devote to any one activity is usually quite short. The satisfaction they experience when they master a new skill is a motivating factor, as is the praise they receive from parents and others. Pressure to perform and high expectations for performance levels not achievable at this age are not in order. Many options for informal and safe gross motor activity, sometimes independent and sometimes with other children, should be provided.

16.B.4 Elementary School Ages

With the cognitive skills achieved by school age, children begin to understand and appreciate games with rules, often, in fact, with a certain amount of rigidity. Many enjoy competition. Organized play, and therefore team sports, becomes possible. Boys and girls at these ages are physically closely enough matched to play team sports together. Attention spans lengthen. Children in the elementary years begin to set and pursue goals which may include the mastery of a sport or sports. These may or may not be sports to which their body characteristics are well matched. For a time, children whose physical development is advanced for their age have a competitive advantage. This advantage may be erased as the development of their peers catches up. After puberty, which occurs at an average age of 10 to 12 for girls and 12 to 14 for boys, males have a weight, height, and strength advantage which results in the subsequent separation of the sexes for many sporting activities.

The role of the involved adult should be to support the child's interests without pressure, to provide a good role model for team participation, to deemphasize winning (children put extreme emphasis there on their own), and to help the child enjoy a number of different sporting activities—for both individual and group participation—so that options are open for a lifetime of enjoyment. Additionally, the adult should assure safe participation by insisting on protective equipment and adherence to rules which prevent injury. These cannot be left to the child.

16.B.5 Young Adolescents

As puberty progresses, the physical disparities among children matched by chronological age or by grade widen (see figure 16-1). Participation in team sports guided by age or grade can become maddeningly frustrating for the late maturer who is at a great weight and height disadvantage. Such a mismatch is thought also to contribute to injury. The understanding of sympathetic parents and coaches may sustain children through this difficult period and guide them to activities in which they can succeed.

Young adolescents (and indeed some older elementary schoolchildren) are capable of demanding training programs and long hours of participation. These are probably reasonable if self-imposed and not demanded and enforced by an adult who is playing out his or her own aspirations, and if

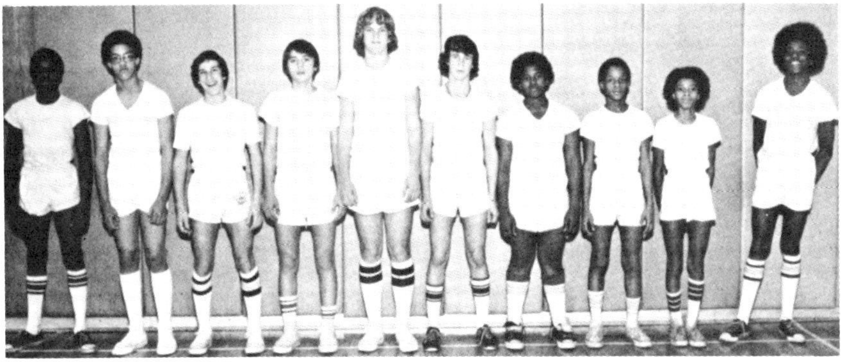

FIGURE 16-1. *Boys in the same eighth-grade physical education class. (From Shaffer 1977. Copyright 1977 by American School Health Association, PO Box 708, Kent, OH 44240. Reprinted by permission.)*

they are balanced by other kinds of activities. However, overuse injuries can result and can cause permanent damage. Pain should be taken seriously and heat illness should be avoided. Exercising children do not adapt well to hot and humid weather and may not recognize the signs of heat stress and the need for frequent water intake (AAP 1982). Some extremely strenuous physical tasks such as long-distance running and weight training may be most appropriately delayed until after puberty when the growth plates of bones have closed and growth-damaging injury is less likely. Sports participation should be carried out in such a way that it enhances rather than interrupts or detracts from the many developmental tasks of the young adolescent.

16.C Opportunities for Protection

STRATEGIES FOR PREVENTING SPORTS INJURIES
(high-priority strategies are indicated by a △)

Selecting Appropriate Sports
△ Match players for size and ability rather than age.
   Delay heavy contact in sports until after puberty.
   Choose sports with child's individual capabilities in mind.
   Avoid some sports altogether.

Changing Practices
   Train and condition players.
   Change rules to prevent impact to the head and neck.
   Ban play for the rest of the game for a participant who has a head injury or

until a complete medical evaluation is made for a player with syncope (fainting/dizziness/passing out).

Changing the Equipment

△ Make equipment safer (e.g., breakaway bases, ski bindings that release).
△ Provide players with protective equipment.

Changing the Conditions of Play

△ Insist on the use of protective equipment.
 Provide trained supervision.
 Eliminate fixed barriers near the field of play.
 Provide energy-absorbing surfaces for walls and playing surfaces.
 Separate players from motor vehicles.

16.C.1 Schools and Child Care Centers

Schools should have established protocols governing sports facilities and activities. Indoor and outdoor facilities should be designed with safety in mind. For example, glass should not be used near playing areas; playing areas should not be contiguous or overlapping and should be surrounded by a buffer zone; protrusions and walls near playing areas should be padded or otherwise protected; problems of moisture, uneven surfacing, etc., should be anticipated and/or remedied when identified (Penman and Niccolai 1985). Only equipment that has been evaluated with safety in mind should be installed and installation should be according to standard specification for that equipment or grade level (ASBO 1986). Facilities and equipment should be inspected regularly. Injury data can help identify hazardous equipment or areas of a facility. Equipment found to be faulty or hazardous should be labeled and removed from use immediately. Trampolines should not be used by schools.

Continual study of new products and standards is necessary to ensure that equipment is as safe as possible and that protective devices and equipment are used when available. Examples of new technologies that may reduce injuries include breakaway bases, face guards, and chest protection for baseball players. Protective equipment should be used in practices as well as games. Types of protective equipment that should be used regularly include eye protection for racquet sports, shin guards for soccer, batting helmets with face shields for baseball, and headgear which protects the ears for wrestlers.

School health-service personnel, physical education teachers, and coaches should work together to ensure proper preparticipation examinations and screening of athletes; to provide effective conditioning and warm-up exercises prior to participation; and to assess the physical environment for suitability for play, such as playing field condition or extreme outdoor temperature which might require eliminating or altering some activities and providing more water than usual. Coaches and physical education teachers and aides should be trained in first aid techniques, and first aid supplies should be available at every practice and game. It is helpful for an individual other than the coach or teacher who is trained to recognize and assess injuries, such as the school nurse or an athletic trainer, to be present at practices and games. Early recognition of injuries can reduce or prevent severe injuries, speed the athlete's return to the sport, and play a part in litigation prevention. A phone and a second adult to make calls should be readily available. The number to call in an emergency should be posted near the phone.

Schools can play a large role in encouraging low-risk sports for all children and in discouraging sports that are inappropriate for young children, such as football (Johnson et al. 1972). Schools should reexamine the value of games in which the goal is to strike a child with an object, such as dodgeball. Rules and regulations for organized and unorganized sports activities should be taught to staff and students. Rules should be evaluated and revised when practices are identified with significant injuries. For example, rule changes in football have been related to a reduction in injuries. Proper procedures must be followed so that skills will be progressive; students should not perform activities for which they are not prepared (ASBO 1986). Procedures should be established to provide for supervision of students arriving before school or early to class (ASBO 1986). The teacher-student ratio should permit close supervision of activities, particularly in gymnastics, where one-on-one spotting has been found to be of value in reducing injuries (Weiker 1985).

Activities that have been suggested as reducing exposure to liability often reduce exposure to physical injury as well. According to a liability checklist developed by Bayless and Adams (1985), coaches and physical educators are advised to (1) point out the foreseeable dangers of participating in an activity in specific terms to students and parents; (2) identify and adhere to all the rules of the game; (3) teach correct technique; (4) supervise with safety in mind; (5) plan and keep records, including parents' and athletes' knowledge of possible injuries, medical exam records, medical clearance from doctors before returning to participation, safety instructions, training rules, cumulative and daily injury reports, and facility checklists; (6) communicate with district administration (school districts should have written administrative policies dealing with athletic safety, including coaches' qualifications and evaluations, standard safety policies, monitoring equipment and facilities for safety, and a mechanism for tracking and recording all injuries); and (7) establish emergency procedures.

Schools can be influential in reducing sports injuries that may occur when school is not in session. For instance, schools can teach children proper techniques for sports activities outside of the usual physical education curriculum. Teaching children the correct way to fall in activities such as skateboarding and roller skating may reduce injuries (Inkelis 1988). Some schools prohibit sports activities considered unsafe, such as skateboarding and riding ATVs or minibikes, on school grounds. School grounds should be evaluated for sources of injury that might occur when school is not in session, such as wires not visible to bicycle riders or rocks or fences that might cause injury to children sledding. These sources should be altered to prevent possible injuries.

Finally, school personnel can collect sports-injury data and use it to effect local policy changes, as the Brookline, Massachusetts, school nurses did. Their collection of data on skateboard injuries occurring outside of school (skateboards were already prohibited on school grounds) was an important factor in the town's banning skateboards on public thoroughfares (Rudisch and Palfrey 1977).

16.C.2 Health Care Providers

To assure healthy sports participation, health care providers must deal with children and sports at both the individual patient and the community level. Health care providers must be prepared to advise patients and their parents on a wide variety of sports-related topics, some of which will be related to healthy development (Is my child old enough? Should I let my child quit the team?) and others to the risk of physical injury (Should my child quit playing basketball because her knees hurt?). The health care provider should be prepared to discuss what is known about the risk of permanent injury or death associated with common sports. There are certain sports which carry such a high risk of catastrophic injury that the health care provider should actually discourage participation—for instance, trampoline use, which has caused a large number of spinal cord injuries for the estimated number of participants, and boxing, which carries a high likelihood of cumulative brain damage. For many sports, the health care provider can counsel use of protective equipment such as helmets. Parents may need to be reminded that buying high-quality equipment (e.g., skis with adequate release systems) is an investment in their child's future. This can be prompted either by a preparticipation physical, by an injury-related visit, or by the answer to the interview questions "What do you like to do for fun? What sports do you play?"

A number of overuse syndromes have been reported in child and adolescent athletes (e.g., Little League elbow, low-back injury with power lifting, stress fractures of the wrist in gymnasts). Health care providers who take care of children should receive enough training in sports medicine to deal with these appropriately or to recognize the need for referral.

Preparticipation sports physicals are a time-honored practice but have not been shown to accomplish what would be highly desirable—to identify the rare child with risk of sudden death during strenuous physical activity due to previously unrecognized cardiac disease (e.g., hypertrophic cardiomyopathy, anomalous origin of the left coronary artery or hypoplastic coronaries, aortic valve stenosis, primary pulmonary hypertension, arrhythmias, prolonged QT syndrome) (Driscoll 1985; Landry 1990). A family history of heart symptoms at an early age or of sudden, unexplained death; a personal history of exercise-related syncope or angina; or physical exam findings suggestive of Marfan syndrome (tall, thin habitus; scoliosis; pectus excavatum; hyperextensive joints; click and murmur of mitral valve prolapse) should prompt further evaluation. Unfortunately, the history and exam do not identify every child at risk. Children with known heart disease may or may not need participation restrictions, based on the nature of their cardiopulmonary dynamics. The advice of a pediatric cardiologist should be sought. Children should not be needlessly restricted. The Committee on Sports Medicine of the American Academy of Pediatrics has provided an updated listing of medical conditions with which a child might need to use special protective equipment or choose less strenuous, noncontact sports (AAP 1988b). Certainly, when contact, collision, and high-impact sports are prohibited, the child should be supported in the choice of any of a number of less risky options. In all cases the preparticipation physical is an opportunity to assess general health, diagnose treatable conditions, conduct an orthopedic screening exam, and provide education about preventing injury, including the use of protective equipment (Landry 1990).

Because of the many team sports which American children enjoy, many health professionals are needed to provide adequate health care input at the community level as team physicians or advisors to organizations sponsoring team sports for children. The high rates of oral injury suggest that a "team dentist" may also be useful (de Wet 1981). Health care providers who serve schools need to attend to the fact that sports participation accounts for the largest proportion of serious school-related injury. A team or school physician or nurse can, of course, evaluate individual injuries but can also provide guidance which will protect the whole team. Specific issues to be emphasized are the safety of the conditions of play (e.g., barriers such as benches removed from the proximity of play, early suspension of play during electrical storms) and the absolutely consistent use of protective equipment (e.g., chest pads for catchers, batting helmets) and rules (e.g., no spearing in football). Prevention of "axial loading," that is, the compression of the cervical spine when the head stops but the body keeps going (Torg 1985) and head injury associated with blows to the head should be among the highest priorities of rules and equipment. Children who suffer head impact severe enough to cause loss of consciousness, confusion which is more than momentary, headache, nausea, vomiting, amnesia, or any neurological sign should not be returned to play. Return-to-play guidelines for a range of injuries are available in a number of sources (AAP 1987; Landry 1990). Adequate skills and equipment for neck stabilization for an injured player should be present at all times, and ready access to a phone assured. Emergency procedures to be used in the event a player collapses or suffers a catastrophic injury should be worked out in advance. Team physicians and nurses must remember that they may be called upon to attend to coaches and spectators, as well. Finally, the health care provider can emphasize the relatively great vulnerability of the child to heat stress

(AAP 1982). Plenty of liquid should be provided before, during, and after participation on a hot day. Water is the fluid of choice (Murphy 1984). The body cools itself by evaporation from the skin, so opportunities for evaporation must be provided—that is, children must be given exercise breaks during which such equipment as helmets and pads are removed.

16.C.3 Public Agencies

Agencies responsible for children's recreation programs should follow the same guidelines outlined for schools and child care centers in section 16.C.1. These guidelines include design and maintenance of facilities, teaching and supervision, and insurance and liability issues.

Community planners and other agencies should provide play areas for children's sports separated from motor vehicle and bicycle traffic and from younger children and pedestrians. Skateboarders should also be separated from traffic. Many of the thousands of children injured annually while skateboarding are youngsters between the ages of 10 and 14 who fall and fracture a bone, but some suffer lethal injury, especially in collisions with motor vehicles. Skateboard parks that have special road surfaces and require protective equipment have been suggested as a way of reducing hazards to pedestrians from skateboarders and to skateboarders from traffic and road surface; however, they may introduce other injuries or increase injury severity (Illingworth et al. 1978). Due to the efforts of health and transportation departments, some communities have banned skateboards on public thoroughfares (Rudisch and Palfrey 1977).

16.C.4 Legislators and Regulators

Legislators and regulators can work to ban hazardous sports equipment, as was successfully accomplished with lawn darts in 1988, when other measures are not enough to prevent serious injury. Sports equipment and protective equipment should be required to meet safety standards. ASTM has published many consensus standards for sports equipment, and the National Operating Committee on Standards for Athletic Equipment (NOCSAE) has established standards for some sports helmets and face guards. The CPSC should act to pass mandatory standards for sports equipment and protective gear not covered adequately by voluntary standards, such as helmets for youth skiers.

16.C.5 Law Enforcement Professionals

Some sports activities, such as skateboarding, may be prohibited in certain locations because they are particularly likely to be hazardous. Law enforcement officers can collaborate with schools and volunteer organizations to foster compliance.

16.C.6 Voluntary Organizations

Communities must provide safe and attractive areas for sports participation (e.g., playing fields for ball, skateboarding courses, and sledding hills all removed by space or barriers from motor vehicle traffic). Sporting areas and facilities need to be well maintained so that they are free of broken glass and defective equipment. In addition, attention must be paid to surface characteristics; surfaces should absorb energy whenever possible (see chapter 15, Playgrounds) and should not be uneven. Impact injuries can be reduced by padding walls and keeping fixed equipment such as benches and drinking fountains far away from the field of play. Good planning, regular maintenance, and adequate supervision reduce injuries and liability.

Groups that sponsor organized sports for children must provide training for adult supervisors which includes prevention of injury, emergency response, and safety equipment. Amateur sports associations can be instrumental in reducing certain types of injuries by requiring the use of protective equipment in all sanctioned games and enforcing compliance, as the Amateur Hockey Association of the United States (AHAUS) did with mouth guards (Castaldi 1986). Such actions should be evaluated for effectiveness and modified as necessary; for example, the AHAUS later mandated full face protection because serious eye injuries continued. Adults in the community must also model safe sports participation including the separation of sports from alcohol consumption.

16.C.7 Designers, Architects, Builders, and Engineers

Arguably the most urgent technology issue for injury prevention in sports is the continued improvement and dissemination of protective headgear. A multipurpose helmet which would adequately protect a child during a number of sporting activities and would be attractive, inexpensive, and easy to maintain would be ideal. Affordable playing surfaces which do not change the enjoyment of the sport but which absorb energy during falls without contributing to lower-extremity injuries are also a priority.

The layout of sporting areas should keep fixed equipment (benches, goalposts, drinking fountains) away from the field of play. Where walls are close, they should be padded. Access to a phone and the ability to bring in emergency vehicles should be assured.

The potential for new designs to cause injury should be considered from the outset. Lawn darts, now banned by the Consumer Product Safety Commission because of their association with penetrating head injury, are an example of a design with an injury risk which might have been anticipated.

A number of specific design issues have been raised which deserve further work, including the following: bimaxillary mouth guards for contact sports; chest protection for child batters; improvement in the catcher's mitt to prevent vascular and nerve damage to the hand and fingers (Medical

World News 1976); eye protection for baseball, racquet sports, and others (Grin et al. 1987); improved protective equipment for ice hockey (Gerberich et al. 1987) and skateboarding (Morgan et al. 1980); evaluation of sled designs which keep the sledder sitting up as a possible solution to head and neck injury and improvement in steering mechanisms for sleds (Landsman et al. 1987); quick-release ski boot-and-binding systems similar to those designed for adults and head protection for child skiers; footwear designs which reduce lower-extremity injury; and wrist guards for skaters (Inkelis et al. 1988).

16.C.8 Business and Industry

Safety equipment should be prominently displayed with other athletic equipment. Industry must make safety sell. More manufacturers of safety equipment are needed. Increased competition will stimulate improvement in designs and more reasonable costs to the consumer.

Manufacturers of sports equipment should be encouraged to offer children's equipment with the same safety features as adults'. For example, manufacturers may not offer the same high-quality ski boot-and-binding release systems for children that they offer to adults. Recent experience in the car industry shows that customers will pay for safety—if sports equipment is designed and marketed with an emphasis on safety, parents may be willing to pay for better quality.

Equipment designed with safety in mind is protective not only for the user, but for the manufacturer as well. Safe equipment reduces the number of injuries and thereby reduces the manufacturer's exposure to product liability.

16.C.9 Mass Media

Children emulate adult heroes, many of whom are sports figures. Good role models can be featured in public-service announcements highlighting prevention of injuries and protective equipment and behavior.

Whenever possible, the media should include the use of safety equipment in sports coverage and applaud its use, thus helping to make it an expected part of the sport—the "thing to wear."

Producers, directors, photographers, artists—all those responsible for creating images of athletes and athletics—can make choices that promote the prevention of sports injury rather than its occurrence.

References

American Academy of Pediatrics. 1982. Climatic heat stress and the exercising child, policy statement. *Pediatrics* 69(6):808–809.

American Academy of Pediatrics. 1983. *Sports Medicine: Health Care for Young Athletes*. Evanston, Ill.: American Academy of Pediatrics.
American Academy of Pediatrics. 1987. *School Health: A Guide for Health Professionals*. Elk Grove Village, Ill.: American Academy of Pediatrics.
American Academy of Pediatrics. 1988a. Infant exercise programs, policy statement. *Pediatrics* 82(5):800.
American Academy of Pediatrics. 1988b. Recommendations for participation in competitive sports, policy statement. *Pediatrics* 81(5):737-739.
Association of School Business Officials International. 1986. *School Safety Handbook*, revised version. Reston, Va.: Association of School Business Officials.
Bayless, MA, and Adams, SH. 1985. A liability checklist. *Journal of PE, Recreation, and Dance*, February, p. 49.
Consumer Product Safety Commission. 1981. *Overview of Sports-Related Injuries to Persons 5-14 Years of Age*. Report prepared by G. Rutherford et al. Washington, D.C.: Consumer Product Safety Commission.
de Wet, FA. 1981. The prevention of orofacial sports injuries in the adolescent. *Int Dent J* 31(4):313-319.
Driscoll, DJ. 1985. Cardiovascular evaluation of the child and adolescent before participation in sports. *Mayo Clin Proc* 60:867-873.
Gerberich, SG, et al. 1987. An epidemiological study of high school ice hockey injuries. *Childs Nerv Syst* 3(2):59-64.
Grin, TR, et al. 1987. Eye injuries in childhood. *Pediatrics* 80(1):13-17.
Illingworth, CM, et al. 1978. 225 skateboard injuries in children. *Clin Pediatr* 17(10):781.
Inkelis, SH, et al. 1988. Roller skating injuries in children. *Pediatr Emerg Care* 4(2):127.
Johnson, CJ, et al. 1972. Injuries resulting in fractures in the Seattle public schools during the school year 1969-70. *J Sch Health* 42(8):454-457.
Kraus, JF, and Conroy, C. 1984. Mortality and morbidity from injuries in sports and recreation. *Ann Rev Public Health* 5:163-192.
Landry, GL. 1990. Sports medicine, in Oski, FA, et al. (eds.): *Principles and Practice of Pediatrics*. Philadelphia: J. B. Lippincott, pp. 919-939.
Landsman, IS, et al. 1987. Injuries associated with downhill sledding. *Pediatr Emerg Care* 3(4):277.
Listernick, D, and Finison, K. 1983. The problem of sports and recreational injuries. *SCIPP Reports* 4(2):1.
Medical World News. 1976. Catchers need more than a mitt: Surgeon says poor protection causes vascular damage. *Medical World News* April 5:77.
Morgan, WJ, et al. 1980. Prevention of skateboard injuries. *Scott Med J* 25(1):39-40.
Murphy, RJ. 1984. Heat illness in the athlete. *Am J Sports Med* 12(4):258-261.
Penman, KA, and Niccolai, FR. 1985. Playing it safe: Designing sports facilities to avoid personal injury and litigation. *American School and University* 57(8):36-38.
Rudisch, GA, and Palfrey, JS. 1977. Skateboard safety, letter. *Pediatrics* 59:953.
Shaffer, TE. 1977. The young athlete. *J Sch Health*, April, p. 222.
Torg, JS. 1985. Epidemiology, pathomechanics, and prevention of athletic injuries to the cervical spine. *Med Sci Sports Exerc* 17(3):295-303.
Weiker, GG. 1985. Club gymnastics. *Clin Sports Med* 4(1):39-43.

Additional Sources of Information

ASTM (Formerly known as the American Society for Testing and Materials)
1916 Race Street
Philadelphia, PA 19103
215-299-5400
   Standards for sports equipment and protective equipment.

National Operating Committee on Standards for Athletic Equipment (NOCSAE)
11724 Plaza Circle
Kansas City, MO 64195
816-464-5470
   Standards for some helmets and face guards.

The Physician and Sportsmedicine
4530 West 77th Street
Minneapolis, MN 55435
   Sports injury statistics resource list (updated annually).

Recreation and Safety Institute (RSI)
PO Box 392
Ronkonkoma, NY 11779
516-563-4800
   Information and consultation on facilities management, staff training, litigation, and legislative trends.

17

Drowning and Other Water-Related Injuries

17.A Facts

Drowning is the major cause of injury mortality in children aged 1-4, and in the 5- to 14-year age-group is surpassed only by motor vehicle–occupant deaths. Drowning rates are highest in 1- to 3-year-old children of both sexes and in teenage males. Each year about 1,500 children under 15 drown; almost half of them are in the 1- to 4-year age-group. The number of near-drownings is not precisely known, but at least 5,000 children are hospitalized for near-drowning annually (Wintemute 1990).

Childhood drowning is an especially serious problem in Alaska, Hawaii, Florida, California, and other southern and western states, in part because of the large number of home swimming pools. (In Alaska the high rates probably reflect extensive reliance on boat transport and very low water temperatures.) Home pools figure prominently in drownings of young children. In Sacramento County, California, they are the site of 58% of all drownings of children younger than 5 years (Wintemute et al. 1987). A common scenario occurs when a toddler falls into a pool while out of sight of any caretaker; often the child is found soon enough that immediate resuscitation attempts would be effective, but resuscitation is not attempted until the rescue squad arrives, often too late. For this reason, it is imperative that anyone who has a swimming pool be trained in cardiopulmonary resuscitation (CPR).

In some states with high drowning rates, swimming pools are less common than in Florida and California. In New Mexico, pool drownings are uncommon, and the majority of toddler drownings involve ditches (such as irrigation ditches) or other small bodies of water near the home (Davis et al. 1985).

Childproof pool fencing that completely surrounds the pool is extremely effective in preventing drowning of young children. Pool barriers that use the residence as one side of the enclosure may reduce access from other yards but not from the home itself. One study found that half of the children who drown in swimming pools in California drown in their own pools (Wintemute et al. 1987); thus, the fencing should separate the pool area from the home and the rest of the yard (see figure 17-1).

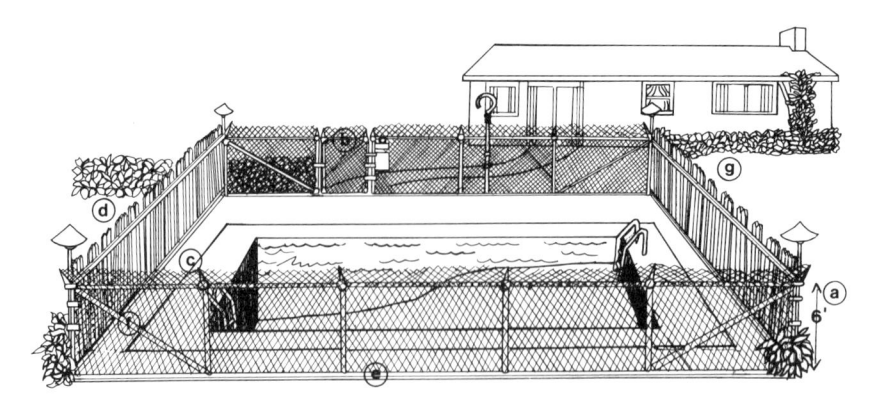

FIGURE 17-1. *Some desirable features of backyard pool fencing, which must surround all four sides of pool. (a) Fencing is at least 6' high; (b) gate is self-closing and locking, with latch near the top; (c) chain linking, if used, has angle extension; (d) other fencing has top that discourages climbing; (e) fencing has continuous footings; (f) framing and braces are on the inside; and (g) periodic gaps in solid fencing allow observation from the outside. (Adapted from CDC 1977.)*

Bathtub drowning is especially likely to involve children with seizure disorders or other young children who have been left unattended. Supporting rings for use in the bathtub with infants can mislead parents into thinking that an infant can be left unsupervised for a short while and have already been associated with deaths. Small amounts of water, as in a diaper pail, ditch, or wading pool, can be fatal to a small child. Particularly hazardous appear to be 3- to 5-gallon "scrub" buckets containing water with cleaning solutions (Scott and Eigen 1980; Walker and Middelkamp 1981).

Suction drains in spas, hot tubs, whirlpool baths, and pools are extremely hazardous, and have proven fatal and caused some injuries to children who have been sucked against the drain or had their hair drawn into the drain so they could not get their faces out of the water. Drain covers, bathing caps, and supervision can help to reduce the risk of trapping children underwater.

Adolescent drowning often involves swimming in unsupervised areas, such as rivers or quarries. Alcohol intoxication is often a factor in teenage drowning; in New Mexico, 40% of the drowning victims aged 15–19 had been drinking (Davis et al. 1985). Undoubtedly, alcohol is involved in some young adolescents' drownings, too. Ironically, there is no evidence to support the widespread belief that children are likely to drown if they swim after eating but ample evidence for the largely unknown fact that alcohol greatly increases the risk of drowning.

There is inadequate evidence for the effectiveness of swimming training in reducing drowning, since such training also has the potential to induce children and adolescents to venture into water that they otherwise might avoid. Similarly, the effectiveness of "drownproofing" and early swimming training for infants in preventing drowning has not been evaluated (Pearn

1985). Training older children in water safety, including life jacket use, may be of greater value. Boating-related drownings most commonly involve older adolescents and adults, but children are sometimes involved. All persons in a boat, children included, should wear a personal flotation device (PFD)—in common parlance, a life jacket.

In addition to drowning, many other injuries are associated with water sports. The most serious are paralyses resulting from diving into shallow water in a pool, river, or other body of water. Propeller injuries to water skiers can also be devastating, and could be eliminated if propellers were adequately shielded. About 4,000 children are injured on swimming pool slides each year; some water slides in amusement parks have caused serious injuries, including injuries to the lumbar spine from pronounced dips in the slide.

17.B Developmental Considerations

17.B.1, 17.B.2, and 17.B.3 Infants, Toddlers, and Preschoolers

Infants cannot swim, nor can they be "waterproofed." They do not have the motor skills for keeping their heads above water nor for getting out of water. They may not be able to maintain their body temperature. They may swallow enough water during a swimming lesson to adversely affect their blood chemistry (Goldberg 1982). This condition, called water intoxication, can lead to seizures, coma, and death. Parents and supervisors of infant water-training programs should adhere to guidelines that limit time in the water as well as other hazards (AAP 1985; ARC 1988).

Infants and toddlers can drown in any collection of water deep enough to cover their noses and mouths. A particularly pertinent example is the drowning of older infants and toddlers in buckets or pails at home. A large bucket partially filled is heavy enough that children can use it to pull to a standing position. If they subsequently fall inside head first, they may not be able to extricate themselves (CPSC 1989). Young children in or around water need constant supervision. An approved flotation device is desirable for children near a pool; inflatable toys will not suffice. Barriers such as fences must separate the unsupervised young child from natural bodies of water near the home and from water hazards on farms.

Infants, toddlers, and even preschoolers, because of their size and strength disadvantages, can be drowned by adults. There are few distinguishing findings in this subtle form of fatal child abuse (Griest and Zumwalt 1989).

17.B.4 Elementary School Ages

By school age many children can swim well enough to keep their heads above water for a short time. Times and distances increase with age and experience. In a study of Australian children, the median age for swimming

10 meters was $6\frac{1}{2}$ (Nixon et al. 1979). Most children swam by age 11. While drowning deaths are relatively infrequent at this age, events that children interpret as posing a serious drowning risk are not. Fifteen percent of primary school students in South Carolina, a state with a relatively high drowning rate (Baker and Waller 1989), reported such a personal incident in the previous year (Schuman 1977).

17.B.5 Young Adolescents

Drowning rates begin to climb again in early adolescence, but only for males. A number of drowning incidents involve boys falling through the ice on lakes, rivers, or ponds. Most warm-weather incidents also occur in rivers, lakes, quarries, or canals rather than at more traditional swimming areas such as pools or beaches. Boating incidents begin to play a larger but still secondary role. Alcohol use apparently contributes to the high rate of drowning deaths among adolescent males. Night swimming with peers and peer pressure may be involved.

17.C Opportunities for Protection

STRATEGIES FOR PREVENTING DROWNING AND
OTHER WATER-RELATED INJURIES
(high-priority strategies are indicated by a △)

Changing the Environment

- △ Surround all sides of home swimming pools with childproof fencing.
- △ Make approved personal flotation devices available on all boats.
    Design spa and pool drains that will not suck in hair or otherwise cause children to be trapped underwater.

Instructing Children in Water Safety

Teach to identify hazardous situations.
Teach to stay afloat.
Increase knowledge of how to use personal flotation devices.
Train in rescue techniques that do not endanger the rescuer.

Changing Adult Behavior

- △ Require all pool owners to receive training in cardiopulmonary resuscitation.
- △ Enforce the use of personal flotation devices by everyone in boats or being towed by boats.
    Teach caretakers never to leave a young child unattended in the bathtub, within reach of a bucket of liquid, or near any body of water deep enough to cover the nose and mouth.

Encourage use of shallow water for infant baths.

Empty pools when they will not be used for an extended period.

17.C.1 Schools and Child Care Centers

Pools, ponds, fountains, and other areas of water at or near schools and child care centers should be inaccessible to children. Several aspects of water safety can be taught to children, including safe rescue techniques, CPR, use and importance of PFDs, and hazard recognition, such as walking on ice and swimming in unsupervised water. Children in rural areas should be taught the dangers of playing in or near irrigation ditches and canals. Education should also emphasize the dangers of combining alcohol use with water activities (Davis et al. 1985; Wintemute et al. 1987).

The effect of teaching all students rudimentary swimming skills has not been adequately evaluated. Some argue that instead of enhancing safety, this may increase risk by causing some inexperienced swimmers to assume risks they otherwise would have avoided.

Swimming pools at schools should be properly marked to indicate water depths, and lifesaving devices should be readily available nearby. Pool doors should be kept locked, no one should be allowed in the pool alone, and teachers on duty should be qualified in lifesaving skills. Children with epilepsy should not be allowed to swim without a lifeguard or competent swimmer being aware of their condition. School swim teams should not permit "hypoxic" training (wherein swimmers hyperventilate and then hold their breath while swimming laps or under water) and should warn of the dangers involved in such training (Orlowski 1988). Schools should encourage the use of their facilities by "adult education" groups such as the Coast Guard Auxiliary or the U.S. Power Squadron for the teaching of boating and waterway safety.

Child care personnel should avoid the drowning hazards of diaper pails and other pails partially filled with cleaning solutions or other liquids. Diaper pails should have conveniently locking lids; other pails should not be left with liquid in them even for a short period of time (Sturner et al. 1976).

17.C.2 Health Care Providers

Physicians should advise all parents to learn CPR and should make a special effort to encourage CPR training for parents who have home pools. All parents should be advised of the need for constant supervision of children around water, about the hazards for small children of even small amounts of water (wading pools, diaper pails, scrub pails, the bathtub, ponds, watering troughs for animals, cattle tanks). Families should be asked about water in their home and recreation environment (including hot tubs) and counseled accordingly. One point of counseling for boaters should be that all persons in a boat should wear a PFD.

Young children should never be left alone in the bathtub! Bath support rings which stick by suction cups to the tub floor cannot be relied on to keep a child's head above water. Drownings have been reported (CPSC 1988a). Supervision should be provided by an adult, not by an older sibling.

Children with epilepsy should not participate in high diving (because of the possibility of a dangerous fall) or competitive underwater swimming. As for all other children, all swimming and water-related activities should be supervised (AAP 1983). Children with epilepsy should swim only in lifeguarded areas or with a competent swimmer who knows of their increased risk—calculated to be four times as high as for children without seizure disorders (Orlowski et al. 1982). Young children with epilepsy should be constantly supervised in the bath. Older patients with epilepsy should bathe in a tub of very shallow water or shower seated with the drain open and a hand-held shower head which will automatically shut off if not pressed (Livingston et al. 1980).

At this time there is no evidence to support recommending infant "swimming" or "water-adjustment" programs. Rare problems have been reported, including fecal contamination of the water and the spread of giardiasis, a parasitic infection of the intestinal tract, and water intoxication without compensatory advantages (AAP 1985). Concerns also include the suspicion that early water training may make children and parents less cautious around water and actually increase drownings. No data yet settle this question.

Emergency medical personnel need special training to react well to immersion injury, including the need for immediate institution of CPR, the benefits of oxygen administration, and the need to consider the possibility that an older child or adolescent was diving and has a spinal cord injury, making neck stabilization mandatory.

Outcome cannot be predicted when a submersion-injured child is pulled from the water. It is crucial that resuscitation be instituted immediately and that the comotose child who responds to vigorous field and emergency department resuscitation receive ultimate care in a pediatric referral center with expertise in neuroresuscitation so that hypoxic brain damage can be minimized (Robinson and Seward 1987).

Drowning can be a difficult-to-detect form of child abuse (see section 17.C.5). A thorough investigation of the circumstances of an infant or toddler drowning in the home is warranted (Griest and Zumwalt 1989).

17.C.3 Public Agencies

Agencies regulating swimming pools and programs for children should follow the same guidelines outlined in section 17.C.1 for schools. Cooperation of agencies and schools regarding facilities and programs is helpful. Agencies can use epidemiological data to identify communities and population groups at greatest risk for drowning; special prevention programs should be targeted to those areas and individuals first.

Agencies can be instrumental in educating the public as to water hazards and water safety through organized public-education campaigns and in the following ways. Cardiopulmonary resuscitation training programs should be targeted to families with small children, particularly those with swimming pools at their homes or nearby (Wintemute et al. 1987). Dangerous locations and irregularities such as holes, dips, or undertows in swimming areas and thin ice should be publicized and clearly marked. Employees who work on or near water should be trained to recognize environmental hazards and to perform emergency rescue techniques (CDC 1988), especially since in several studies children submerged for long periods of time or apparently dead at the time of rescue recovered following resuscitation efforts (Siebke et al. 1975; Pearn 1977). Appropriate warning systems and evacuation plans for natural disasters involving water (hurricanes, floods, etc.) should be established and publicized.

Supervised swimming areas should be established if lacking. Standardized procedures concerning lifeguards should be established, including training programs and guard-to-swimmer ratios. Lifeguards should be taught current CPR techniques, and those guarding areas of deep water might be trained in deep-water resuscitation techniques, found to be successful in Australia (Manolios and Mackie 1988).

Hazardous unsupervised swimming areas should be made inaccessible. Barriers should be constructed to separate children from water, including sites such as riverbanks, bridges, wharfs, and ditches. Guardrails should protect child passengers and other occupants from drowning due to motor vehicle immersion. Air bags and seat belts, which help prevent head injury, may prevent drowning subsequent to the driver's loss of consciousness (Wintemute et al. 1987), and should be required. Agencies working with rural or farm families should promote the use of barriers to separate children from ponds, irrigation ditches, troughs, and other sources of water.

Agencies can require licensing for public, private, and semiprivate (e.g., apartments, condos) pool, spa, and hot tub construction and ownership based on safety requirements. All pools should conform to the guidelines presented in section 17.C.7, particularly as regards pool fencing.

CPR training should be mandatory for residential pool and spa owners. Accessible lifesaving devices should be required.

Agencies should restrict the sale and consumption of alcohol in areas used for recreational boating and swimming (CDC 1988). Boaters suspected of being intoxicated should be tested for alcohol levels, and stiff penalties should be given to those found boating while intoxicated. Authorities should enforce these policies, as well as other safe-boating policies, such as wearing PFDs and observing speed limits in boats. Minimum age restrictions can be set for operating power boats and personal watercraft (individual power boats that look like snowmobiles). Personal watercraft operators should be required to wear USCG-approved PFDs. Water-skiers should also be required to wear approved PFDs, and observers should be required on tow boats.

Agencies can establish standards for water slide and amusement park water rides (such as the guidelines for construction and use of water slides developed by the South Australian Health Commission) (Radford and Baggoley 1987). Some examples of measures to reduce injuries are installing starting gates and traffic lights, "giving attendants greater control over sliders and the means to communicate with them," providing adequate space between sliders, and installing safe drain covers to prevent entrapment.

Protective-service and health agencies should educate families about the hazards of drowning in bathtubs, in diaper pails and buckets, in the farm setting, and in other hazardous local sites. Protective-service workers must be alert to the occurrence of intentional drowning incidents and should cooperate with other investigating authorities (see section 17.C.5).

17.C.4 Legislators and Regulators

Suggestions for state and local regulations concerning pool, spa, and hot tub design, construction, and ownership are given in section 17.C.3. Four-sided pool fencing is an intervention likely to be very effective; it should be a priority for legislators and regulators in areas with many swimming pools. Voluntary standards exist for safety covers for pools, spas, and hot tubs (see section 17.C.7). Design and/or performance standards should be developed for fencing, gates, and associated hardware (Wintemute 1990). Local lawmakers should also consider requiring CPR training for residential pool owners.

Legislators and regulators should be concerned with the regulatory aspects outlined in section 17.C.3 for farm safety, keeping alcohol out of water recreation areas, and water slide safety. Safe boating and waterskiing policies are discussed in section 17.C.3. Federal regulations require that a USCG-approved PFD be carried for every person on board a recreational boat (USCG 1973). Voluntary standards exist for various aspects of many types of boats. Jurisdiction over the conduct of boaters will vary according to the type of waterway. Local authorities should contact state and federal authorities (e.g., the U.S. Coast Guard) so that intergovernmental cooperative efforts regarding waterway safety will be possible.

17.C.5 Law Enforcement Professionals

Law enforcement officers are crucial to the enforcement of federal, state, and local regulations concerning water and boating safety. As possible first responders, police, fire, parks, and other enforcement personnel need to achieve and maintain skills in CPR, including those for infants and young children. Selective enforcement of speed and alcohol laws has been successful in reducing boating-related deaths and injuries. Other boating policies are discussed in section 17.C.3. Boating and water safety courses sponsored by law enforcement departments can be valuable in raising awareness of water hazards and safe boating practices.

When drowning deaths occur in the home, police should investigate the scene, determine who was supervising, and obtain a thorough history. Such deaths sometimes result from child maltreatment or deliberate submersion (Brooks 1988; Perrot and Nawojczyk 1988). Intentional drowning must be considered when a young child is discovered unconscious but wet after an apparent delay in summoning help and when a neonate is found in a toilet (Griest and Zumwalt 1989). Detection may protect other children in the home.

17.C.6 Voluntary Organizations

Organizations can push for well-enforced domestic swimming pool safety regulations for their own communities. Many studies suggest that fencing regulations for domestic pools will greatly reduce the number of child drownings (Wintemute 1990). Community-based organizations can also be active in identifying appropriate families and educating them about water hazards in the area, providing adequate and accessible rescue equipment and personnel, and encouraging and sponsoring CPR training for all adolescents and adults. Organizations should eliminate unsupervised water hazards for small children, such as filled buckets or bathtubs and large aquaria, from their own activity areas if they serve families.

A number of voluntary organizations provide swimming or boating training for children. Such organizations should ensure that the facilities they use are safe and well run, that safety rules oriented to the special needs of children of various ages are devised and enforced, that supervision is adequate and includes persons experienced in CPR, that appropriate rescue equipment is present, and that emergency procedures are developed in advance of need. Particularly important is insistence on the use of a PFD by everyone in a boat. Additionally, medical histories—particularly whether or not children have a seizure disorder—are pertinent, although supervision should not be relaxed even when no children in the group have such a history. Additional issues of importance to voluntary organizations providing water-based activities are outlined in other sections of this chapter; detailed guidelines can be obtained from the YMCA and the American Red Cross.

17.C.7 Designers, Architects, Builders, and Engineers

Fencing height for backyard pools should subvert most climbers and therefore should be at least 5 feet and preferably 6 feet high, surrounding all four sides of the pool, with a self-closing and locking gate with a latch near the top. Chain linking should have an angle extension; other fencing should have tops that discourage climbing. Fencing should have continuous footings or be imbedded in the earth at least 6 inches; framing and braces should be on the inside rather than the outside to prevent unauthorized entry; and fences should allow observation from the outside (CDC 1977) (see figure 17-1). Fencing for on-surface and portable pools should be as stringent as for in-ground pools—the drowning hazard is just as real. Voluntary standards exist for pool covers (ASTM 1989) which are helpful when a pool will not be used for an extended period. Pool covers require repeated action, however, so they are not as effective as more automatic measures such as fencing. Pool alarms also exist that sound when an object (such as a wandering toddler) enters the pool, but problems with false alarms or failure to alarm have been reported, so the designs can be improved (Wintemute 1990). In addition, someone must remember to activate the alarm when the pool is to be unoccupied. Pool covers and alarms are not acceptable substitutes for fencing. Pools to be equipped with diving boards require rigorous attention to such features as board length, depth of the water at plummet, distance to upslope, pool length, and distance to overhead structures (CPSC 1985). Diving injuries most often affect older adolescent and young adult males, so are not addressed comprehensively here. At least 4,000 pediatric injuries each year are associated with pool slides, suggesting opportunities for design and placement improvements.

Drainage systems for pools, spas, and hot tubs should be designed so that pipes are too small to admit a child's body. Children's abdomens or other body parts can become attached by suction to a hot tub or spa drain outlet, causing entrapment and immersion injury. Elevated grates can be retrofitted on older spas with single outlets. New spas should have two suction outlets and grates (Monroe 1982). Long hair can become entangled in the drainage system and hold a child's head underwater. Drainage systems and grates must be designed to prevent this occurrence (CPSC 1988b). Water slides must also be designed to prevent entrapment (CDC 1986) and other injuries (see Section 17.C.3).

Highly visible swimwear may make submerged swimmers easier to see (Dietz and Baker 1974). Personal flotation devices that are more comfortable than current designs might be worn more regularly. Ski belts (narrow beltlike life preservers) are comfortable for water-skiers and other users but do not keep an unconscious or exhausted person from a face-down position, as USCG-approved Type I, II, and III PFDs do. Disabled water skiers have drowned while wearing ski belts (Hummel and Gainor 1982); the design should be revised. Other waterskiing injuries could be prevented if boat propellers were thoroughly shielded.

When artificial bodies of water are used to enhance a building or its grounds, the drowning hazard to children should be recognized and minimized. Likewise, childproof barriers should divide children from natural bodies of water in busy public places where many children are likely to escape supervision.

17.C.8 Business and Industry

Products that present a clear drowning risk for children, such as spas and home pools, should be marketed with explicit warnings and with installation instructions designed to minimize risk.

Businesses that make pools, spas, and water slides available to the public should honor the strictest possible safety standards, build in the most automatic protection possible, and take a leadership role in helping the public to enjoy their products without injury.

New products that may present a hazard should undergo premarket testing and careful monitoring for associated injuries once released to the market. Children are unlikely to be able to use personal watercraft (tiny power boats) safely but may be capable of operating them. Marketing that attracts child users should be avoided, and purchasers should be warned that the products are inappropriate for child use.

17.C.9 Mass Media

A number of crisp messages are available to augment drowning prevention through the mass media, including the following: even swimmers drown, children can drown at home, PFDs are important, pools should be fenced on four sides, children should be supervised constantly around water, and CPR should be started immediately should a drowning occur. A public-awareness campaign which underscored drowning hazards and drowning prevention in Australia helped to reduce childhood immersion injury (Nixon et al. 1986). The link between drowning and boating mishaps and alcohol may not be as well recognized by the public as the link between automobile injury and alcohol. Intoxicated parents are unable to supervise children appropriately, and many adolescents who drown have been drinking. While preventing drowning will require much more than simply pointing this out, building public awareness of the relationship between drowning and alcohol is in order.

Reports of drowning can be accompanied by strategies for prevention. As is the case for pedestrian and other types of injuries, investigative reporters may point out drowning patterns within a community. Awareness of patterns may lead to remediation of environmental hazards or public knowledge of safe practices.

Boaters should be portrayed, whenever possible, wearing PFDs, and an implicit connection between alcohol consumption and water sports should be avoided.

References

American Academy of Pediatrics. 1983. Sports and the child with epilepsy, policy statement. *Pediatrics* 72(6):884–885.
American Academy of Pediatrics. 1985. Policy statement: Infant swimming pro-

grams, in *Policy Reference Guide*. Elk Grove Village, Ill.: American Academy of Pediatrics, p. 270.

American Red Cross. 1988. *American Red Cross Infant and Preschool Aquatic Program, Instructor's Manual*. Washington, D.C.: American Red Cross.

ASTM. 1989. Emergency standard performance specifications for safety covers and labeling requirements for all covers for swimming pools, spas and hot tubs. Standard ES 13-89, in *1989 Annual Book of ASTM Standards*, Volume 15.07, End Use Products. Philadelphia: ASTM.

Baker, SP, and Waller, AE. 1989. *Childhood Injury: State-by-State Mortality Facts*. Baltimore: Johns Hopkins University Injury Prevention Center.

Brooks, JG. 1988. Near drowning. *Pediatrics in Review* 10(1):5–10.

Centers for Disease Control. 1988. Drownings in the United States, 1978-1984. *MMWR CDC Surveill Summ* 37(1):27–33.

Centers for Disease Control (CDC). 1986. Fatality at a waterslide amusement park—Utah. *MMWR* 35(26).

Centers for Disease Control. 1977. "Kidproofing" the backyard pool. Today's Health, Dept. of Health, Education, and Welfare Publication No. (CDC) 77-8336.

Consumer Product Safety Commission. 1985. *National Pool and Spa Safety Conference*. Washington, D.C.: Consumer Product Safety Commission and National Spa and Pool Institute.

Consumer Product Safety Commission. 1988a. *CPSC Warns of Drowning Hazard with Baby "Supporting Ring" Devices*. Consumer Product Safety Alert. Washington, D.C.: Consumer Product Safety Commission.

Consumer Product Safety Commission. 1988b. *Four Children Drown and More Are Injured from Hair Entrapment in Drain Covers for Spas, Hot Tubs, and Whirlpool Bathtubs*. Consumer Product Safety Alert. Washington, D.C.: Consumer Product Safety Commission.

Consumer Product Safety Commission. 1989. Large buckets are drowning hazards for young children. *Safety News* August. Washington, D.C.: Consumer Product Safety Commission.

Davis, S, et al. 1985. Drownings of children and youth in a desert state. *West J Med* 143(2):196–201.

Dietz, PE, and Baker, SP. 1974. Drowning: Epidemiology and Prevention. *Am J Public Health* 64:303.

Goldberg, GN, et al. 1982. Infantile water intoxication after a swimming lesson. *Pediatrics* 70(4):599–600.

Griest, KJ, and Zumwalt, RE. 1989. Child abuse by drowning. *Pediatrics* 83(1):41–46.

Hummel, G, and Gainor, BJ. 1982. Waterskiing-related injuries. *Am J Sports Med* 10(4):215–218.

Livingston, S, et al. 1980. Drowning in epilepsy. *Ann Neurol* 7(5):495.

Manolios, N, and Mackie, I. 1988. Drowning and near-drowning on Australian beaches patrolled by life-savers: A 10-year study, 1973-1983. *Med J Aust* 148(4):165–167, 170–171.

Monroe, B. 1982. Immersion accidents in hot tubs and whirlpool spas. *Pediatrics* 69(6):805–807.

Nixon, J, et al. 1986. Fifteen years of child drowning—a 1967-1981 analysis of all fatal cases from the Brisbane Drowning Study and an 11 year study of consecutive near-drowning cases. *Accid Anal Prev* 18(3):199–203.

Nixon, J, et al. 1979. Swimming ability of children: A survey of 4000 Queensland children in a high drowning region. *Med J Aust* 2(5):271-272.

Orlowski, JP. 1988. Adolescent drownings: Swimming, boating, diving, and scuba accidents. *Pediatr Ann* 17(2):125.

Orlowski, JP, et al. 1982. Submersion accidents in children with epilepsy. *Am J Dis Child* 136(9):777-780.

Pearn, J. 1985. Current controversies in child accident prevention: An analysis of some areas of dispute in the prevention of child trauma. *Aust NZ J Med* 15: 782.

Pearn, J. 1977. Neurological and psychometric studies in children surviving freshwater immersion accidents. *Lancet* Jan 1: 7.

Perrot, LJ, and Nawojczyk, S. 1988. Nonnatural death masquerading as SIDS (sudden infant death syndrome). *Am J Forensic Med Pathol* 9(2):105-111.

Radford, AJ, and Baggoley, C. 1987. Waterslide accidents in South Australia. *Aust Fam Physician* 16(11):1664-1667.

Robinson, MD, and Seward, PN. 1987. Submersion injury in children. *Pediatr Emerg Care* 3(1):44-49.

Schuman, SH, et al. 1977. Risk of drowning: An iceberg phenomenon. *J Am Coll Emerg Physicians* 6:139-143.

Scott, PH, and Eigen, H. 1980. Immersion accidents involving pails of water in the home. *J Pediatr* 96(2):282-284.

Siebke, H, et al. 1975. Survival after 40 minutes' submersion without cerebral sequelae. *Lancet* 1:1275-1277.

Sturner, WQ, et al. 1976. Accidental asphyxial deaths involving infants and young children. *J Forensic Sci* 21(3):483-487.

United States Coast Guard. 1973. Personal Flotation Devices. 33 *CFR* 175.

Walker, S, and Middelkamp, JN. 1981. Pail immersion accidents. *Clin Pediatr (Phila)* 20(5):341-343.

Wintemute, GJ, et al. 1987. Drowning in childhood and adolescence: A population-based study. *Am J Public Health* 77(7):830-832.

Wintemute, GJ. 1990. Childhood drowning and near-drowning in the United States. *Am J Dis Child* 144:663-669.

Additional Sources of Information

American Red Cross (ARC)
National Headquarters
2025 E Street, NW
Washington, DC 20006
202-728-6531
   Water safety instruction materials.

National Drowning Prevention Network (NDPN)
PO Box 161661
Fort Worth, TX 76161
817-236-3430
   Newsletter featuring drowning-prevention issues.

National Safe Boating Council
U.S. Coast Guard Headquarters
Commandant (G-BBS)
Washington, DC 20593
202-267-0994
   Materials for National Safe Boating Week, information on boating safety regulations and classes and PFDs.

National Swimming Pool Safety Committee
c/o Consumer Product Safety Commission
5401 Westbard Avenue
Washington, DC 20207
301-492-6580

Information on child drownings and diving safety, including annual Operation Waterwatch public awareness program.

Parents of Near Drowning (POND)
c/o Maureen Ryan
1375 Box Canyon Road
San Jose, CA 95120

Support group for parents, with chapters around the United States.

YMCA of the United States
101 North Wacker Drive
Chicago, IL 60606
217-977-0031

Guidelines for swim programs.

CONCLUDING REMARKS: A CALL TO ACTION

Children are our most precious commodity, providing joy today and hope for the future. Keeping them safe and whole in body and mind is of the greatest importance. Fortunately, responsibility for protecting them from injury does not rest on parents alone. Decision makers have important means to keep children from being hurt or killed; this book has detailed a wealth of such opportunities.

The task ahead is lighter because it is shared, but it will not be accomplished if we assume that someone else will do it. Using this book, leaders in many fields can identify ways they themselves can address the problem. For the reader who wishes to stimulate others to take action, local data and case histories will be invaluable. We now have a good understanding of most aspects of childhood injury on a national level, but your greatest power comes when you can bring statistics to life with personal touches and close-to-home examples. Conversely, if the evening news captures the tragedy of another childhood drowning or fatal house fire, the moment is ripe to provide reporters and community leaders with detailed information on the size and cause of the problem and how it can be solved.

Our greatest strength comes from the knowledge that many injuries can be prevented, that children need not be subjected to disability, that childhood death from injury often reflects a failure to apply existing knowledge and technology. Exciting, lifesaving opportunities await the decision makers to whom this book is addressed.

APPENDIX

Selected Sources of General Information about Childhood Injury Prevention

American Academy of Pediatrics
Committee on Injury and Poison
 Prevention
141 Northwest Point Boulevard
PO Box 927
Elk Grove Village, IL 60009
800-433-9016

American National Standards
 Institute (ANSI)
1430 Broadway
New York, NY 10018
212-354-3300

American Red Cross
National Headquarters
2025 E Street, NW
Washington, DC 20006
202-728-6531

American Trauma Society
1400 Mercantile Lane
Suite 188
Landover, MD 20785
800-556-7890

ASTM (formerly known as the
 American Society for Testing and
 Materials)
1916 Race Street
Philadelphia, PA 19103
215-299-5400

Bioengineering Center
Wayne State University
818 West Hancock
Detroit, MI 48202
313-577-1347

Center for Injury Prevention
Building One, Room 306
San Francisco General Hospital
San Francisco, CA 94110
415-821-8209

Centers for Disease Control
Division of Injury, Epidemiology, and
 Control
Center of Environmental Health and
 Injury Control
Atlanta, GA 30333
404-488-4646

Child Accident Prevention Foundation
 of Australia
26 Liverpool Street
Suite 5
Melbourne 3000, Victoria
Australia

Child Accident Prevention Trust
28 Portland Place
London W1N 4DE
England

Communities for Child Safety
National 4-H Council
7100 Connecticut Avenue
Chevy Chase, MD 20815
301-961-2822

Consumer Federation of America
1424 16th Street, NW
Washington, DC 20036
202-387-6121

Consumer Product Safety Commission
National Injury Information Clearinghouse
5401 Westbard Avenue
Washington, DC 20207
800-638-CPSC or 301-492-6424

Consumer's Union of the United States
256 Washington Street
Mt. Vernon, NY 10553
914-667-9400

Harborview Injury Prevention and Research Center (HIPRC)
Harborview Medical Center
325 Ninth Avenue, ZX-10
Seattle, WA 98104
206-223-3408

Injury Prevention Center at Harvard University
Harvard School of Public Health
677 Huntington Avenue
Boston, MA 02115
617-732-1080

Injury Prevention Research Center
University of Alabama at Birmingham
UAB Station/THT 433
Birmingham, AL 35294
205-934-7845

Injury Prevention Research Center
University of North Carolina
CB #3430
Chapel Hill, NC 27599
919-962-2202

Johns Hopkins Injury Prevention Center
The Johns Hopkins School of Public Health
624 North Broadway
Baltimore, MD 21205
301-955-3995

Juvenile Products Manufacturers Association, Inc.
66 East Main Street
Moorestown, NJ 08057
609-234-9155

National Maternal and Child Health Clearinghouse
Bureau of Maternal and Child Health and Resources Development
Public Health Service
U.S. Department of Health and Human Services
38th and R Streets, NW
Washington, DC 20057
202-625-8410

National Safe Kids Campaign/National Coalition to Prevent Childhood Injury
111 Michigan Avenue, NW
Washington, DC 20010
202-939-4993 or 202-338-7227

National Safety Council
444 North Michigan Avenue
Chicago, IL 60611
312-527-4800

National Spinal Cord Injury Association
600 West Cummings Park
Suite 2000
Woburn, MA 01801
800-962-9629 or 617-935-2722

New England Network to Prevent Childhood Injuries/
Education Development Center, Inc.
55 Chapel Street
Newton, MA 02160
800-225-4276 or 617-969-7100

Occupational Safety and Health
 Administration (OSHA)
U.S. Department of Labor
200 Constitutional Avenue, NW
Room N3101
Washington, DC 20210
202-523-8576

Snell Memorial Foundation
PO Box 493
St. James, NY 11780
516-862-6545

Statewide Comprehensive Injury
 Prevention Program (SCIPP)
Department of Public Health
Division of Family Health Services
150 Tremont Street
Boston, MA 02111
617-727-1246

Toy Manufacturers Association
200 Fifth Avenue
Suite 740
New York, NY 10021
212-675-1141

UCLA Injury Prevention Research
 Center
School of Public Health
University of California, Los Angeles
Los Angeles, CA 90024
213-825-7066

United States Coast Guard
Commandant (G-NAB)
2100 Second Street, SW
Washington, DC 20593
202-267-0994

INDEX

N.B.: Numbers in italics refer to illustrations and tables.

Accident-proneness, 6–7
Acetaminophen, 106, 182
Activated charcoal, 108
Adolescents, ix. *See also* Young adolescents
Advertising. *See* Mass media
Air bags, 15, 32, 36, 40, 41; and drowning, 223
Alcohol: and advertising, 25; and drowning and other water-related injuries, 218, 220, 221, 223, 224–25, 227; and motor vehicle occupants, 32, 35, 37; and pedestrians, 63; and poisoning, 102; and sports, 213; and suicide, 173, 180
Amateur Hockey Association of the United States, 213
American Academy of Pediatrics: bicycle size guidelines of, 71; first aid recommendations for choking child, 118; recommendations for carrying children on bicycles, 74; sports participation recommendations, 211
American Association of Poison Control Centers, 100, 105, 107
American Horse Show Association, 141
American Red Cross, water safety guidelines of, 225
Amusement parks, water slides in, 219, 224
Animal-related injuries, 140–48; and dog bites, 140, 141–42, 144, 146; and farm animals, 141, 142, 144, 146; and horseback riding, 141, 142, 144, 145–46, 146–47; and morbidity, 140, 141; and mortality, 140, 141; and poisoning, 104, 106; and prevention strategies, list of, 142–43; and rabies, 141, 144, 145, 146; and safety education, 143, 144, 145; and sources of additional information, 148
ANSI standards, 23; for bicycle helmets, 68–69
Architects. *See* Designers, architects, builders, and engineers
Asphyxiation. *See* Choking and suffocation
Aspiration. *See* Choking and suffocation
Aspirin, 8, 100, 105, 182
Assaults, 4–6, 161–71; and burns, 90, 91, 92, 93–94; and choking and suffocation, 114, 115, 119, 120, 121; and drowning, 219, 222, 224, 225; and falls, 128, 132–33; and firearms, 149, 151; and morbidity, 162; and mortality, 162; and nonviolent conflict-resolution training, 165, 168; and poisoning, 101, 104–5; and prevention strategies, list of, 164; recognizing and reporting, 162, 165, 165–66, 167; and scalds, 86, 87; sources of additional information on, 169–71; by strangers, 161; and suicide, 172, 174. *See also* Discipline
ASTM standards, 23; for equestrian helmets, 141, 145–46; for sports equipment, 212
ATVs, 46, 47–48, 53; ban on three-

ATVs (*continued*)
  wheeled, 47–48, 50, 53; legislation on, 48, 51, 52; standards for, 51–52, 53
Automatic protection. *See* Prevention strategies

Balloons, 112, 123–24; standards for, 112, 117, 120
Bathtubs: and drowning, 218, 222, 224; and falls, 135
Batteries: and choking, 122; and poisoning, 107
Bicyclist injuries, 68–82; and bicycle size guidelines, 71; and bike paths and roadways, 74–75, 77, 78, 195; and carrying children as passengers, 70, 73–74, 75; conspicuity, 68, 73, 75–76, 78; and morbidity, 68; and mortality, 68, 69; and prevention strategies, list of, 71–72; and safety education, 72, 74, 76, 77; sources of additional information on, 81–82. *See also* Helmets
Bleachers, 131, 136
Boating. *See* Drowning: and boating
Body measurements (anthropometry), 190
Bottle bills, 127, 134
Builders. *See* Designers, architects, builders, and engineers
Building/housing codes, 22; and choking, 120; and falls, 133, 136, 180; and fires and burns, 91, 92, 94
Bunk beds: and choking and suffocation, 113, 122; falls from, 127, 134, 135
Bureau of Alcohol, Tobacco, and Firearms, 154–55
Burns. *See* Fires and burns
Business and industry: and animal-related injuries, 146; and assaults, 168; and bicycle injuries, 79–80; and choking and suffocation, 123; and drowning and other water-related injuries, 227; and falls, 136; and firearm injuries, 157–58; and fires and burns, 95–96; and motor vehicle occupant injuries, 41; and other motorized vehicle injuries, 48, 53; and pedestrian injuries, 65; and playground injuries, 199; and poisoning, 108; and sports injuries, 214; and suicide, 182; and toy-related injuries, 157–58
Business and industry, role of, in injury prevention, 23

Campaigns, health-promotion: to increase bicycle helmet use, 69, 75, 76–77; to prevent drowning, 227; to prevent motor vehicle occupant injuries, 36, 38, 40, 41; to prevent pedestrian injuries, 65
Carbon monoxide: and poisoning, 102, 103; and suicide, 181
Cardiac disease and sports preparticipation exams, 210–11
Cardiopulmonary monitors, 37, 91, 91–92, 95
Cardiopulmonary resuscitation (CPR) training, 90, 217, 221, 223, 224, 225
Car safety seats, 29–30, 33, 40, 41; and booster seats, 31, *31*, 34; and car beds, 37, 40; legislation on, 31–32, 38–39, 133; and low-birthweight infants, 33, 36–37, 40; misuse of, 30, 36, 39, 40; options for children who've outgrown, 31; rear- vs. forward-facing, 30, 33; rear- vs. front-seat position for, 30, 33, 36; rental programs for, 37, 38, 39–40, 41. *See also* Motor vehicle occupants
Caustic Poisons Act of 1927, 105
Centers for Disease Control (CDC) guidelines for suicide clusters, 179
Changing tables, 131, 135
Child abuse. *See* Assaults
Child development and injury, ix. *See also specific age groups*
"Children Can't Fly" fall-prevention program, 10, 128
Child-resistant packaging, 9, 104, 105–6, 107, 108
Choking and suffocation, 111–26; and balloons, 112, 117, 120, 123–24; and cave-ins, 114, 115, 118, 121; and coins, 122; and cribs, 112–13, *114*, 122; defined, 111; first aid and safety education for, 117; and foods, 111–12, 117, 118, 123–24; and garage doors, 114, 115, 119, 122–23; inten-

tional, 114, 115, 119, 120, 121; and mortality, 111, 112; and prevention strategies, list of, 116–17; and refrigerators and other appliances, 113–14, 115, 118, 120, 121, 121–22, 124; sources of additional information on, 125–26. *See also* Furniture and equipment; Suicide and suicide attempts; Toys

Cigarette lighters, 85, 93

Cigarettes, firesafe, 85, 93, 95, 96

Coal gas and suicide, 182

Coalitions to prevent injury, 18, 19, 20, 21

Community planners. *See* Public agencies

Consumer Product Safety Commission: and the business community, 23; reporting to, 17, 119; and *Safety News*, 117. *See also* Standards

Corporal punishment. *See* Discipline

Cribs: and choking and suffocation, 112–13, *114*, 122; and falls, 127, 129, 131–32; standards for, 113, 117, 120–21

Crush injuries, 111, 115, 128, 131

Day care. *See* Public agencies; Schools and child care centers

Dealers. *See* Business and industry

Death rates. *See* Mortality

Dentists: and motor vehicle occupants, 37; and sports, 211. *See also* Health care providers

Designers, architects, builders, and engineers: and animal-related injuries, 145–46; and assaults, 168; and bicycle injuries, 77–79; and choking and suffocation, 122–23; and drowning and other water-related injuries, 225–26; and falls, 134–35; and firearm injuries, 156–57; and fires and burns, 53, 94–95; and motor vehicle occupant injuries, 40–41, 95; and other motorized vehicle injuries, 53, 95; and pedestrian injuries, 64–65, 196–97; and playground injuries, 196–99; and poisoning, 107–8; and sports injuries, 213–14; and suicide, 182

Designers, architects, builders, and engineers, role of, in injury prevention, 21–22

Discipline: and assaults, 6, 161–64, 165, 166, 167, 168; and burns, 87; and suicide, 175

Drowning and other water-related injuries, 217–30; and bathtubs, 218, 222, 224; and boating, 219, 220, 223–24, 224–25, 227; in buckets, 218, 219, 221, 224; and diving, 219, 222, 226; epilepsy and, 218, 221, 222, 225; intentional, 219, 222, 224, 225; and morbidity (near-drowning), 217; and mortality, 4, 217; and prevention strategies, list of, 220–21; snowmobiles and, 47; sources of additional information on, 229–30; and water safety training/"drownproofing," 218–19, 221, 222, 225; and waterskiing, 219, 224, 226; and water slides, 219, 224, 226. *See also* Pools and spas

Elderly people: and fires and burns, 94; and stair falls, 136

Elementary school ages: and animal-related injuries, 140, 142; and assaults, 163–64; and bicycle injuries, 70–71; and choking and suffocation, 115; defined, ix; and drowning and other water-related injuries, 219–20; and falls, 129; and firearm injuries, 151; and fires and burns, 88; and motor vehicle occupant injuries, 34; and other motorized vehicle injuries, 49; and pedestrian injuries, 59; and playground injuries, 192; and poisoning, 102, 103; and sports injuries, 192, 206; and suicide, 115, 174–75

Elevators: and choking and suffocation, 114, 115, 123; and falls, 129, 134

Emergency medical care, 7, 11; for choking and suffocation, 115; for drowning and other water-related injuries, 222, 225; for fires and burns, 92, 93; for horseback-riding injuries, 143, 146; for injuries resulting from farm machines and other motorized vehicles, 51, 52; for motor vehicle occupants, 37; for sports injuries, 211. *See*

Emergency medical care (*continued*) *also* Cardiopulmonary resuscitation (CPR) training; First aid
Enforcement, primary and secondary, 19, 31–32, 39
Engineers. *See* Designers, architects, builders, and engineers
Entrapment. *See* Choking and suffocation
Environmental Protection Agency (EPA), 106

Falls, 127–39; in bathtubs, 135; from bleachers, 131, 136; and glass, 127, 131, 134, 208, 213; from furniture, 127, 128, 132, 133, 134, 135 (*see also* Furniture and equipment); and intentional injuries, 128, 132–33; and mortality, 127; and prevention strategies, list of, 130; and snow and ice, 133; sources of additional information on, 139; from windows, 10, 127, 129, 131, 136; and window guards, 128, 133, 134. *See also* Playgrounds; Stairs
Family violence: 86, 93, 155–56, 166, 167. *See also* Assaults
Farms: and choking and suffocation, 114, 115, 118, 119, 120, 122; and drowning and other water-related injuries, 219, 221, 223, 224; and falls, 136; and fires and burns, 88; and machine-related injuries, 46, 48–49, 50, 51, 53–54; and poisoning, 106, 107. *See also* Animal-related injuries; Urban/rural differences
Federal Hazardous Substances Act, 105
Federal Insecticide, Fungicide, and Rodenticide Act, 106
Fetus as motor vehicle occupant, 33
Firearms, 149–60, 161; and hunting injuries, 150, 156; and inflicted injuries, 149, 151; mistaken for toys, 149–50, 151, 154, *157*, 157–58; and mortality, 3, 4, 149, *150*; nonpowder, 150, 151, 153, 155; and prevention strategies, list of, 151–52; as public health problem, 153–54, 158; risk of injury from, vs. protective value of, 150, 152; and safe-storage practices, 153, 156, 157; and safety training, 152, 156; Second Amendment and, 153; sources of additional information on, 159–60. *See also* Suicide and suicide attempts; Toys
Fire departments: and fires and burns, 90, 92; and poisoning, 106
Fire escapes: and falls, 129; and fires and burns, 91, 92
Fires and burns, 85–99; and arson, 85, 88, 92, 94; and cardiopulmonary monitors, 91–92, 95; and chemical burns, 107–8; and cigarette lighters, 85, 93; and clothing ignition and flame-retardant materials, 85, 87, 93, 94–95; and contact burns, 86, 87, 95; and electrical burns, 86, 87, 88, 91, 95, 96; and fire escapes, 91, 92; and fire extinguishers, 91, 92, 93; and fire-safe cigarettes, 85, 93, 95, 96; and fireworks, 86, 88, 93, 94, 96; and house fires, 4, 85, 92, 96; and intentional injuries, 86, 87, 88, 90, 91, 92, 93–94; and morbidity, 86; and mortality, 4, 85; and prevention education, 90, 94; and prevention strategies, list of, 88–89; and smoke detectors, 85, 91, 92, 93, 94, 96; and smoke inhalation, 85, 95; sources of additional information on, 98–99; and sprinkler systems, 85, 91, 92, 94, 95, 96; and vaporizers, 10, 91, 92. *See also* Scalds
Fireworks. *See* Fires and burns: and fireworks
First aid: for choking and suffocation, 117, 118, 119, 124; for fires and burns, 90, 91, 96; for poisoning, 103–4, 106 (*see also* Syrup of ipecac); for sports injuries, 209. *See also* Cardiopulmonary resuscitation (CPR) training; Emergency medical care
Furniture and equipment: and choking and suffocation, 118, 122; falls from, 127, 128, 132, 133, 134, 135, 136. *See also* Bunk beds; Changing tables; Cribs; High chairs; Infant cushions; Playpens; Stair gates; Strollers; Walkers; Water beds

Garage doors, 114, 115, 119, 122-23
Gas Appliances Manufacturers' Association, 95-96
Geographical differences, 4; and drowning, 217; and farm-machine injuries, 48; and house fires, 85. *See also* Urban/rural differences
Giardiasis, 222

Handicapped children: and choking and suffocation, 112; and drowning and other water-related injuries, 218, 221, 222, 225; and fires and burns, 89; as motor vehicle occupants, 36, 37, 40; and playgrounds, 194, 196; and poisoning, 107; and sports participation, 211
Health care providers: and animal-related injuries, 143; and assaults, 165-66; and bicycle injuries, 73-74; and choking and suffocation, 118-19; and drowning and other water-related injuries, 221-22; and falls, 128, 132-33; and firearm injuries, 153; and fires and burns, 91; and motor vehicle occupant injuries, 36-37; and other motorized vehicle injuries, 50-51, 74; and pedestrian injuries, 61-62; and playground injuries, 194; and poisoning, 103, 104-5; and sports injuries, 208, 210-12; and suicide, 119, 176, 177-79
Health care providers, role of, in injury prevention, 16-17
Health departments. *See* Public agencies
Helmets: baseball, 204, 208; equestrian, 141, 145-46, 146-47, 204-5; multipurpose, 135, 213; skiing, 205, 212
Helmets, bicycle, 68-69, 74, 77-78, 80; campaigns to increase use of, 69, 75, 76-77; legislation on, 75, 76; schools' role in promoting, 16, 72-73
Helmets, motorcycle and other motorized vehicle, 46, 47, 48, 50, 51, 52, 54
High chairs: and choking and suffocation, 122; falls from, 127, 129, 131, 132, 134, 135
Home health visits to prevent assaults, 166

Homicide. *See* Assaults
Hospitals: and choking and suffocation, 119; and falls, 132; and motor vehicle occupant injuries, 37; and suicide, 177, 179
Hospitals, role of, in injury prevention, 16

Infant cushions, 112, 117, 122
Infants: and animal-related injuries, 140, 141-42; and assaults, 162-63, 168; and bicycle injuries, 70, 73-74; and choking and suffocation, 112, 114-15, 142; defined, ix; and drowning and other water-related injuries, 218, 219, 222; and falls, 128, 132; and firearm injuries, 151; and fires and burns, 86-87; and motor vehicle occupant injuries, 33; and other motorized vehicle injuries, 49; and pedestrian injuries, 57-58; and playground injuries, 191; and poisoning, 101, 107; and sports injuries, 205; and suicide, 174
Infants, low-birthweight, and car safety seats, 33, 36-37, 40
Injury: defined epidemiologically, 7; sources of additional information on, 11-13
Injury Prevention: Meeting the Challenge, 18
Insurance industry: and fires and burns, 92, 95; and motor vehicle occupants, 41. *See also* Business and industry
Intent: spectrum of, 4-5; in suicide, 172
Intentional injury. *See* Assaults; Suicide and suicide attempts

Kerosene: and house fires, 85, 92; and poisoning, 100, 106

Labeling: for flame-retardent materials, 95; for foods, 112, 123; for furniture and equipment, 136; for grain bins, 122; for motorized vehicles, 53; for playground equipment, 199; for poison prevention, 101, 105, 107, 108; for toys, 112, 119, 120, 122, 123; for water heaters, 96

Latchkey (self-care) children: and fires and burns, 90–91; and standards for adult supervision, 92, 93, 96
Law enforcement professionals: and animal-related injuries, 145; and assaults, 20, 167–68; and bicycle injuries, 76; and choking and suffocation, 121; and drowning and other water-related injuries, 224–25; and falls, 134; and firearm injuries, 155–56; and fires and burns, 93–94; and motor vehicle occupant injuries, 38, 39; and other motorized vehicle injuries, 52; and pedestrian injuries, 63–64; and playground injuries, 196; and poisoning, 106; and sports injuries, 212; and suicide, 134, 181
Law enforcement professionals, role of, in injury prevention, 20
Lawn darts, 212, 213
"Learn Not to Burn" burn prevention curriculum, 90
Legislators and regulators: and animal-related injuries, 144–45; and assaults, 19, 167; and bicycle injuries, 75–76; and choking and suffocation, 120–21; and drowning and other water-related injuries, 224; and falls, 127, 133–34; and firearm injuries, 154–55, 180; and fires and burns, 86, 92–93; and motor vehicle occupant injuries, 31–32, 38–39, 133; and other motorized vehicle injuries, 46, 48, 51–52; and pedestrian injuries, 62–63; and playground injuries, 195–96; and poisoning, 103, 105–6; and sports injuries, 212; and suicide, 180
Legislators and regulators, role of, in injury prevention, 19
Liability, 6; and choking and suffocation, 123; and playgrounds, 195, 196; and sports, 209, 212, 213, 214
Life Safety Code, 22
Litigation as prevention strategy, 10

Manufacturers. *See* Business and industry
Marketing. *See* Business and industry; Mass media

Marketing, social, role of, in injury prevention, 24. *See also* Mass Media
Mass media: and animal-related injuries, 146–47; and assaults, 169; and bicycle injuries, 74, 80; and choking and suffocation, 123–24; and drowning and other water-related injuries, 227; and falls, 136–38; and firearm injuries, 158; and fires and burns, 96; and motor vehicle occupant injuries, 16, 41–42; and other motorized vehicle injuries, 54; and pedestrian injuries, 65; and playground injuries, 199–200; and poisoning, 108; and sports injuries, 214; and suicide, 108, 173, 181, 182–83
Mass media, role of, in injury prevention, 23–25
Minibikes. *See* Motorized vehicles other than cars
Mopeds. *See* Motorized vehicles other than cars
Morbidity, 3; and animal-related injuries, 140, 141; and assaults, 162; and ATVs, 47; and bicycle injuries, 68; and drowning and other water-related injuries, 217, 219; and farm-machine injuries, 48; and horseback-riding injuries, 141; and motorcycle injuries, 46; and motor vehicle occupant injuries, 29; and other motorized vehicle injuries, 47; and nonpowder firearm injuries, 150; and pedestrian injuries, 57; and playground injuries, 189; and poisoning, 100; and scalds, 86; and snowmobile injuries, 47; and sports injuries, 203, *204*
Mortality: and animal bites, 140; and assaults, 162; and bicycle injuries, 68, *69*; and choking and suffocation, 111, 112; and drowning and other water-related injuries, 4, 217; and falls, 127; and farm-machine injuries, 48; and firearm injuries, 3, 4, 149, *150*; and horseback-riding injuries, 141; and house fires, 4, 85; and motorcycle injuries, 46; and motor vehicle occupant injuries, 3, 4, 29, *30*, 42; and pedestrian injuries, 57, *58*; and poisoning, 100; and sports injuries, 203; and sui-

cide, 4, 114, 172; and war, compared with motor vehicle occupant deaths, 42. *See also* Geographical differences; Racial differences; Sex differences; Socioeconomic status; Urban/rural differences
Mortality, injury, 3; by cause, *5*; compared with other causes, *4*; source of data on, 18
Mothers Against Drunk Driving (MADD), 19
Motorcycles. *See* Helmets; Motorized vehicles other than cars
Motorized vehicles other than cars, 46–56; and burns, 53, 88, 95; and choking and suffocation, 113; and farm machines, 46, 48–49, 50, 51, 53–54; licensing of, 46, 47, 52; and injury prevention strategies, list of, 50; and minibikes, 46, 47; and mopeds, 46, 47, 50, 51; and morbidity, 46, 47, 48; and mortality, 46, 48; and motorcycles, 46, 51–52; and snowmobiles, 46, 47, 50, 51, 113; sources of additional information on, 55–56. *See also* ATVs; Helmets
Motor vehicle occupants, 29–45; and air bags, 15, 32, 36, 40, 41; and burns, 95; and drowning, 223; and falls, 133; and injury prevention strategies, list of, 35; and morbidity, 29; and mortality, 3, 4, 29, *30*, 42; rear- vs. front-seat position of, 30, 31, 32, 33, 36, 38, 41; restraints and behavior of, 34; and roadway design, 32–33, 40, 41; and safety education, 36, 37, 156; school buses and, 36; side-impact protection of, 29–30, 37, 40; sources of additional information on, 44–45; and speed of vehicle, 32, 39, 41; and vehicle design, 32, 39, 40. *See also* Car safety seats; Seat belts
Munchausen Syndrome by Proxy, 105

National Association of Home Builders' National Research Center, 94
National Center on Child Abuse and Neglect, 162; National Incidence Study of, 162, 163
National Committee for Prevention of Child Abuse, 166–67, 168
National Fire Protection Association, 22, 90
National Highway Traffic Safety Administration, 61
National Operating Committee on Standards for Athletic Equipment, 212
Natural disasters and drowning, 223
Near-drowning, 217
Neglect, 4, 6, 161; and car safety seats, 6, 30, 38; and falls, 133; and fires and burns, 86, 93; and poisoning, 101; and standards for adult supervision, 92, 93, 96; and suicide, 174. *See also* Assaults
Nonpowder firearms, 150, 151, 153, 155

Obstetricians, 37. *See also* Health care providers

Pacifiers, 112, 113, 117, 119
Parental supervision as prevention strategy, 8
Parents Anonymous, 168
Pedestrians, 57–67; age of, for independent street crossing, 61–62; and conspicuity, 57, 64, 65; and injury prevention strategies, list of, 60–61; and morbidity, 57; and mortality, 57, *58*; and right turn of vehicle on red signal, 63; and safety education, 58, 59, 61; and school buses, 61, 63–64, 64–65; sources of additional information on, 67
Personal Flotation Devices (PFDs), 219, 224, 226, 227
Personal freedom, 10, 19
Pharmacists and poisoning, 104, 106
Play, developmental stages of, 190–92
Playgrounds, 189–202; design guidelines for, 190, 195–96, 197–98; and falls, 129, 134, 189, 198; and hanging/entrapment, 122, 190, 197–98; and injury prevention strategies, list of, 192–93; and morbidity, 189; public vs. home, 189; surfacing for, 189–90, 193, *198*, 198, 199; sources of additional information on, 201–2

Playpens, 112, 113, 117, 122
Poison-control centers, 100, 103–4, 107, 108; standards for, 105
Poisoning, 6, 8–9, 100–110; and acetaminophen, 106, 182; and aspirin, 8, 100, 105; and batteries, 107; carbon monoxide, 102, 103, 181; and child-resistant packaging, 9, 104, 105–6, 107, 108; intentional, 101, 104–5; kerosene, 100, 106; prevention strategies, list of, 102–3; and medications, 100, 103, 104, 105, 106, 107; and morbidity, 100; and mortality, 100; and preventive education, 101, 103, 105; and smoke inhalation, 85, 95; sources of additional information on, 109–10; and syrup of ipecac, 101, 104, 107, 108; and veterinary products, 104, 106. *See also* Suicide and suicide attempts
Poison Prevention Packaging Act, 104, 105–6, 108, 145
Pools and spas, 217, 222, 223, 227; and alarms and covers, 226; CPR training for owners of, 221, 223, 224; and drains, 218, 226; and fencing, 217, *218*, 224, 225–26, 227; and guidelines for schools, 221; and pool slides, 219, 226. *See also* Drowning and other water-related injuries
Preschoolers: and animal-related injuries, 141–42; and assaults, 163; and bicycle injuries, 70; choking and suffocation, 115; defined, ix; and drowning and other water-related injuries, 219; and falls, 129, 136; and firearm injuries, 151; and fires and burns, 87; and motor vehicle occupant injuries, 34; and other motor vehicle injuries, 48, 49; and pedestrian injuries, 59; and playground injuries, 191–92, 194; and poisoning, 102; and sports injuries, 205–6; and suicide, 174
Prevention programs, design and evaluation of, 18
Prevention strategies, 7–10; automatic, 8–9, *9*; in relation to event, 7, *8*; and spectrum of intent, 6
Prevention strategies, list of: for animal-related injuries, 142–43; for assaults, 164; for bicycle injuries, 71–72; for choking and suffocation, 116–17; for drowning and other water-related injuries, 220–21; for falls, 130; for firearm injuries, 151–52; for fires and burns, 88–89; for injuries related to motorized vehicles other than cars, 50; for motor vehicle injuries, 35; for pedestrian injuries, 60–61; for playground injuries, 192–93; for poisoning, 102–3; for sports injuries, 207–8; for suicide, 175–76
Protective equipment: for fires and burns, 90; for horseback riding, 146; required for certain medical conditions, 211; for sports, 204–5, 208, 212, 213–14; for users of motorized vehicles other than cars, 46, 47, 51, 53. *See also* Helmets
Puberty, 206, 207
Public agencies: and animal-related injuries, 144; and assaults, 166–67; and bicycle injuries, 74–75; and choking and suffocation, 119–20; and drowning and other water-related injuries, 222–24; and falls, 133; and firearm injuries, 153–54; and fires and burns, 91–92; and motor vehicle occupant injuries, 38; and other motorized vehicle injuries, 51; and pedestrian injuries, 62, 195, 212; and playground injuries, 194–95; and poisoning, 105; and sports injuries, 212; and suicide, 176, 177, 179–80
Public agencies, role of, in injury prevention, 17–19

Racial differences, 4; and falls, 127; and suicide, 172
Radar detectors, 39, 41
Recalls, 23; of car safety seats, 41; and choking and suffocation, 119, 123, 124; of motor vehicles other than cars, 53
Refrigerators. *See* Choking and suffocation
Rehabilitation, 7, 11
Risk-management systems, 195

Scalds: and hot liquids, 86, 87, 89, 95; intentional, 86, 87, 92; and morbidity, 86; and tap water/water heaters, 6, 86, 87, 91, 91–92, 94, 95–96

School buses: and motor vehicle occupants, 36; and pedestrians, 61, 63–64, 64–65; and poisoning, 103

Schools and child care centers: and animal-related injuries, 143; and assaults, 15, 164–65; and bicycle injuries, 72–73, 210; and choking and suffocation, 117–18; and drowning and other water-related injuries, 221; and falls, 130–32; and firearm injuries, 152–53; and fires and burns, 89–91; and motor vehicle occupant injuries, 35–36, 156; and other motorized vehicle injuries, 50, 210; and pedestrian injuries, 61 (*see also* School buses); and playground injuries, 193–94; and poisoning, 103–4; and sports injuries, 15, 208–10, 211; and suicide, 103, 176–77, 180

Schools and child care centers, role of, in injury prevention, 14–16

Seat belts, 16, 30–31, *32*, 34, 40, 41; automatic, 32, 40, 41; campaigns to increase use of, 24, 38, 40, 41–42; and drowning, 223; legislation on, 31–32, 38–39, 133; primary enforcement of laws governing, 31–32, 39; and school buses, 36; use of, during pregnancy, 33. *See also* Motor vehicle occupants

Sex differences, 3–4; and animal-related injuries, 140, 141; and assaults, 163; and bicycle injuries, 68; and body measurements (anthropometry), 34, 190; and choking and suffocation, 114; and drowning and other water-related injuries, 217; and falls, 129; and firearms, 3, 149; and fires and burns, 85, 87; and motor vehicle occupant injuries, 3, 29; and nonpowder firearm injuries, 150; and pedestrian injuries, 57; and playground injuries, 189; and poisoning, 100; and sports injuries, 203, 206; and suicide, 172

Snell helmet standards: for bicycle, 68–69; for horseback riding, 141

Snowmobiles. *See* Motorized vehicles other than cars

Socioeconomic status, 4; and assaults, 4, 162; and choking and suffocation, 114; and house fires, 4, 85

South Australian Health Commission, 224

Sports injuries, 203–16; and baseball, 203, 204, 208; and basketball, 203; and boxing, 210; and football, 203, 204, 205; and golf, 203; and heat stress, 207, 211–12; and hockey, 203, 213; and morbidity, 203, *204*; and mortality, 203; and overuse, 207, 210; and preparticipation exam, 208, 210–11; and prevention strategies, list of, 207–8; and return to play guidelines, 204, 211; and rules and injury prevention, 204, 209, 211; and safe environment/conditions of play, 205, 208–9, 211, 213; and skateboarding, 209–10, 212; and skiing, 205, 214; and sledding, 131, 210, 214; sources of additional information on, 216. *See also* Animal-related injuries; Drowning and other water-related injuries; Helmets; Protective equipment

Stair gates: and choking and suffocation, 113, 122, 135; and falls, 129, 132, 134–35; standards for, 117

Stairs: and choking and suffocation, 120, 131, 135–136; design considerations for, 130–31, 135–36, *137*; and falls, 127, 128, 129. *See also* Stair gates

Standards, 23; for adult supervision, 92, 93, 96; for ATVs, 51–52, 53; for bicycle helmets, 68–69, 76, 77–78; for bleachers, 136; for boats, 224; and choking, 123; for cigarette lighters, 93; for cribs, 113, 117, 120–21; for crib toys, 120; for equestrian helmets, 141, 145–46; for firearms, 155; for flame-retardant materials, 93, 94–95; for furniture, 136; for garage-door openers, 122–23; for home heating, 92; for motor vehicles, 39, 40; for motorized vehicles other than cars, 47, 51–52, 53; for pacifiers, 112; for play-

Standards (*continued*)
  ground equipment, 195–96; for playpens, 117; for poison-control centers, 105; for pool covers, 226; for refrigerators, 113–14, 121; for school buses, 63; for small parts (toys), 112, 117, 120; for sports equipment, 212; for stair gates, 117; for stairs, 136; for toy guns, 158; for walkers, 133; for water slides, 224
Strangulation. *See* Choking and suffocation
Strollers, 131
Students Against Drunk Driving (SADD), 153
Substance abuse: and assaults, 167; and poisoning, 102; and suicide, 172, 175. *See also* Alcohol
Suffocation. *See* Choking and suffocation
Suicide and suicide attempts, 172–85; clusters of, 176–77, 179; and depression, 101, 173, 175, 177–78; with firearms, 149, 172, 173, 180, 181, 182; and gestures, 173, 182; by hanging, 114, 115, 119, 172, 181; imitative, 173, 175, 181, 182–83; by jumping, 129, 179; and mortality, 4, 172; by poisoning, 100, 103, 172, 178–79, 181, 182; and prevention programs, 176, 179, 180; and prevention strategies, list of, 175–76; risk assessment of, 178; sources of additional information on, 185; and survivors, 179–80; and treatment, 178; warning signs of, and risk factors, 172, 177, 178
Syrup of ipecac, 101, 104, 107, 108

Toddlers: and animal-related injuries, 141–42; and assaults, 163; and bicycle injuries, 70; and choking and suffocation, 115, 129; defined, ix; and drowning and other water-related injuries, 217, 219, 226; and falls, 128–29, 136; and firearm injuries, 151; and fires and burns, 87; and motor vehicle occupant injuries, 33–34; and other motorized vehicle injuries, 48, 49; and pedestrian injuries, 58; and playground injuries, 191; and poisoning, 101, 103; and sports injuries, 205–6; and suicide, 174
Toys: and choking (small parts), 112, *113*, 119, 120; and crib toys, 113, 120, 122; and falls, 132; and firearms, 151, 155, 157, *157*; and motor vehicles, 41; and toy boxes, 113. *See also* Nonpowder firearms; Standards
Tractors. *See* Farms: and machine-related injuries
Trampolines, 194, 199, 203, 208

Uniform Vehicle Code: and bicyclists, 75; and motor vehicle occupants, 38–39
Urban/rural differences, 4; and falls, 127; and house fires, 92; and injuries related to motorized vehicles other than cars, 52; and pedestrian injuries, 57. *See also* Geographical differences
U.S. Pony Club, 141

Violence prevention programs: and firearm injuries, 154, 156; and nonviolent conflict-resolution training, 152, 165, 168
Voluntary organizations: and animal-related injuries, 145; and assaults, 168; and bicycle injuries, 76–77; and choking and suffocation, 121–22; and drowning and other water-related injuries, 225; and falls, 134; and firearm injuries, 156; and fires and burns, 94; and motor vehicle occupant injuries, 39–40; and other motorized vehicle injuries, 52; and pedestrian injuries, 64; and playground injuries, 196; and poisoning, 106–7; and sports injuries, 213; and suicide, 107, 181
Voluntary organizations, role of, in injury prevention, 20

Walkers: and burns, 87; and falls, 127, 128, 132, 135, 138; standards for, 133
Water beds, 117
Water intoxication, 219, 222
Werther effect (imitative suicide), 183
"Willie Whistle" pedestrian education program, 61

YMCA water safety guidelines, 225
Young adolescents: and animal-related injuries, 142; and assaults, 164; and bicycle injuries, 71; and choking and suffocation, 115; defined, ix; and drowning and other water-related injuries, 218, 220; and falls, 129; and firearm injuries, 151; and fires and burns, 88; and motor vehicle occupant injuries, 34–35; and other motorized vehicle injuries, 46, 49, 88; and pedestrian injuries, 59–60; and playground injuries, 192; and poisoning, 102, 103, 105, 106; and sports injuries, 192, 206–7; and suicide, 102, 105, 114, 115, 129, 149, 172, 175

Zoning regulations. *See* Legislators and regulators; Public agencies